Kevin AND *Me*

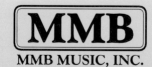

MMB

MMB MUSIC, INC.

CONTEMPORARY ARTS BUILDING
3526 WASHINGTON AVENUE
SAINT LOUIS, MISSOURI 63103-1019 USA
314 531-9635; 800 543-3771 (USA/Canada); Fax 314 531-8384
http://www.mmbmusic.com

To my precious children, Kevin and Megan...each of whose presence helped me to move forward in my healing. My love for them motivated me to go past my fears, to have the courage to be strong, and to keep on believing in miracles.

*K*evin AND *Me*

Tourette Syndrome and the Magic Power of Music Therapy

PATRICIA HEENAN

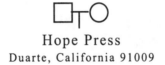

Hope Press
Duarte, California 91009

Kevin and Me

by

Patricia Heenan

~

Published by
Hope Press
P.O. Box 188,
Duarte, CA 91009

For other books, visit our website at **www.hopepress.com**
See order form on back leaf

Library of Congress Cataloging-in-Publication Data

Heenan, Patricia, 1943-
    Kevin and me : tourette syndrome and the magic power of music therapy : a mothers story / Patricia Heenan.
        p.   cm.
    Includes index.
    ISBN: 1-878267-02-7
    1. Heenan, Kevin—Health.   2. Tourette syndrome—
Patients—United States—Biography.   3. Music therapy.
I. Title.
RC375.H44   2000
362.1'9683—dc21   00-57243
[B]   CIP

Printed in the U.S.A.

Contents

With appreciation to our music therapist Hope Young and my niece Julia Bourland for inspiring me to share my story.

With love to my devoted friend Brad Caffey for his inspiration, technical assistance, and dramatic editing.

With gratitude to my caring friend Nona Kean for cheering me on while helping me edit my book.

With loving regards to my dear friend Beverly Griggs for encouraging me to tell my story and assisting me with editing.

With thanks to my two friends Rodney Cunningham and Peggi Purcell for their gift of photography.

With love and acknowledgement to Teresa Wingfield and my daughter Megan for contributing to the artistry of the book.

With a huge "thank you" to all of the people who have helped me with Kevin through the years.

Preface

I sincerely wish to share the true story of Kevin and me to inspire all of you parents to believe in your own authority and to advocate for your children. I encourage you to stay committed to your loved ones and to engage very closely in your children's lives. My son's improvement has resulted from my deep involvement in his life and my continual search to find ways to support him. I have bravely ridden through Kevin's developmental stages, his fluctuating symptoms of Tourette syndrome, and his behaviors of ADHD, OCD, and conduct disorder. In his twenties, music therapy helped him to deal with his control issues and taught me to flow with his unpredictable behaviors.

In describing Kevin's past and his recovery through music therapy, I hope to enthuse Touretters and their family members, psychologists, teachers, and medical professionals to explore music therapy as a medium for re-organizing the brain and influencing healthy behaviors. Since music therapy is gaining acceptance in mainstream medical circles, its services are available in private centers and in school districts through their special education department.

After consulting with neurologists and other specialists for fifteen years, I found music therapy to be the key to unlocking Kevin's heart. The use of music created the bridge to reaching the core of my son, gently calming his Tourette syndrome and assisting him to open up. Since I loved music, I jumped at the opportunity to participate in music therapy sessions with him.

In therapy, Kevin and I bonded in a safe, controlled environment and allowed peaceful music to restore him and our troubled relationship. We communicated with each other through a mirroring technique, playing musical instruments, singing, and other forms of expression. The therapeutic effects of music touched our souls at a deep level and enabled me to see who my son really was, beneath his confusing disorder. Kevin, now twenty-nine, continues to benefit from the therapy's soothing effects in his own individual sessions.

As a result of our music therapy, we have a loving, safe relationship and work side by side in volunteer jobs. Serving as Kevin's job coach, I have passionately pursued job opportunities for him. On the job, his motivation feeds from the synergy that we created in our music therapy sessions. I will continue to serve as his anchor until he can work without supervision.

Writing my story has been a powerful healing event for me. Being the mother of a son with a severe behavioral disability, I have experienced the whole range of emotions from despair and frustration to laughter and joy. In revealing traumas, I have released deep-seated emotions that have helped me to heal wounds and strengthen myself. I hope that some of the intense scenes in this book will comfort you and your loved ones with Tourette, who may identify with similar traumatic experiences. I also hope our success will inspire and uplift you.

I believe that we are equipped as helpers to meet the challenges of caring for children with neurological imbalances. I also believe we have purposeful lessons to learn from these children, who are serving us in our own healing process.

1

Narrow Escape

My sixteen-year-old son is yelling in my face, "F%@# you!!!" while charging at me in the corner of the kitchen. Suddenly my fear propels me to get both of us in the car. I hide my tears, for I'm afraid he might see how vulnerable I feel. Putting up a tough front, I assure myself he won't physically hurt me. And even though he's already hurt me many times before, I silently cry to myself, *He won't hurt me again!* Maybe the drive to my office will divert him, and he'll forget that I'm his target.

In the car he seems calm and quiet. I heave a sigh of relief and catch my breath. I arrive at the office and walk backwards up the steps. I barely reach the door before I'm flung against its edge. *Ouch!!!* And now the nightmare is coming true! For months I've been haunted with the fear of his hurting my head. Escaping for my life, I flee from my first-born as he chases me down the street. Out of breath, I seek refuge in a small church. I desperately convey my need to the minister's wife to leave him there for awhile.

Frantically returning home without my son, I inquire about admission into an adolescent unit at a private hospital. I find out that, because of his age, he must sign himself in. Again I am stricken with fear! Am I stuck with an out-of-control son who only sees me as a target?! How can I make him sign himself in? Surely I can trick him into signing the papers. A thousand more questions flood my brain: *Will he ever leave me alone? Will I ever get my life back? Why does he hate me? Did I do anything wrong? What have I done to create this? Will he ever respect and love me? Why is this happening to me? Have I done enough? Is it time for me to give up? Can I trust the hospital to take good care of him? Will this be a better place for him to live? Am I running away from my job as a parent?*

Actually, I took Kevin to the hospital and he signed himself in. Even though he didn't understand what was happening, he surrendered. He stayed in the adolescent unit for two months until his psychiatrist placed him in a treatment center. He didn't like the hospital and refused to participate at all. At least, it provided a safe environment for him, and my home was safe again. Grief-stricken, I cried for months and began to recover from the insanity in my life.

2

Background Check

Author's note: This chapter gives a brief overview of my life with Kevin, highlighting significant events during our twenty-nine years together. The following chapters will delve into these events with more detail.

When Kevin was born, he was a beautiful, healthy-looking baby. However, by age four, his broken sentences indicated a delay in his language development. Two months before he was six years old, he started making bizarre grimaces and bodily gestures. A strange condition took hold of my boy, like a sudden intruder. Our pediatrician diagnosed him with Tourette syndrome, a neurological disorder of hyperactivity and involuntary facial and motor tics. A medication called Haldol was able to control his facial and motor tics, improve his speaking fluency, and suppress bouts of anxiety.

After Kevin turned six, his father and I divorced. For four years Kevin lived with my daughter and me. At ten, my boy fell into a web of the complexities of Tourette syndrome with its associated disorders, displaying temper tantrums, hallucinations, and aggressive behaviors. On account of these behaviors and the need for testing, I placed him in a children's psychiatric unit at the state hospital, where he surprisingly lived for three years. Although the separation anxiety that he experienced drastically altered his personality, he was still not well enough to live at home.

When Kevin was thirteen, he was transferred to a youth center for two years. Participating in sports at the center helped him to develop focus, to build self-esteem, and to work out his distress. He was fortunately endowed with an athletic body that enabled him to excel in swimming, touch football, and his favorite sport basketball.

Following his discharge from the center, Kevin lived with his Dad for nine months and, before his sixteenth birthday, moved to my house for seven long months. I was on constant duty—night and day! During these teenage years, his TS condition worsened when he manifested compulsive behaviors and the baffling *coprolalia*—a symptom involving involuntary outbursts of obscene words and socially inappropriate remarks.

Unfortunately, the drug Haldol was not able to control his anger attacks toward me nor his compulsive behaviors of talking inappropriately to people, staring overtly at strangers, or childishly running away from home. Kevin's dark wavy hair, big brown eyes, and beautiful smile gave him such a handsome appearance that his obscene finger gestures out in public took people by surprise. His anger grew, and after a narrow escape I frantically separated from him and placed him in a private hospital for two months. Following my son's brief time there, he went to live at a treatment center for six months.

Kevin's speaking disability progressed in his teens to severe difficulty in answering questions. Stressed and confused, he commonly responded by saying, "I don't know." His slow language development hindered him; after many years of IQ testing, he was labeled *mildly retarded* as a result of his low verbal scores. Finally, at the age of seventeen, he began living in boarding homes until an appropriate group home opened up for him two years later.

In his early twenties, he became plagued with unwanted thoughts that he vocalized incessantly to me and others during frequent compulsive spells. His periodic obscene words and emotional outbursts demanded the need for on-going supervision. Kevin's friendliness motivated him to talk, but unfortunately his strange language confused people. Since Kevin didn't look disabled, strangers were politely disgruntled if he pointed a finger at them and made remarks, such as "You are devil," or "You are God." His favorite expressions were "I am good," and "I am bad." When Kevin considered himself bad, I sometimes wondered if negative forces resided within him that told him he was bad. He appeared ambivalent, struggling to find himself between his two parts.

During this same period Kevin frequently ran away from home and school searching for sodas. (His runaways for sodas earned him the nickname "Soda Man Running.") Under risperidone—a medication that inhibited his runaways and powerfully quelled his emotional outbursts—a sweet personality began to blossom at age twenty-three and warm my heart.

At this point, I would like to share a little history about myself that prepared me for my later adventures with Kevin. Born into an obstetrician's family, I heard my father receive medical emergency calls at all hours of the night. During the evening, I frequently took his calls before he came home. I also saw him deal with minor emergencies and unexpected events that required immediate attention. Later in life, as the student judge of a self-governing dorm system in a girls' college, I was exposed to inappropriate behaviors and thus gained experience for future dealings with my son's emotional problems. As an adult, I taught English as a second language at the local university for ten years and later worked as the enrollment director for personal growth seminars for four years. Teaching foreign students gave me practice communicating without words on an intuitive level. I was able to transfer my intuitive approach to my interactions with Kevin. Unknowingly, my past gave me experience handling the emotional and physical challenges of raising Kevin.

Five years ago, Kevin became more in tune with himself through the magic of music therapy. During sessions his verbal and physical tics subsided for longer periods. Over time, he learned that he had the power to control his impulses if he chose to; thus, he transformed from a violent man into a more peaceful person.

Faced with a language disability, Kevin responded remarkably to the music therapy process, which stimulated his right brain and enabled him to smile and express himself more. In turn, his higher functioning right brain strengthened his left brain's ability to communicate. As a result, he began initiating conversations more readily and answering questions without too much hesitation.

Music therapy helped me to understand my son's disorder. As a co-client, I joined in Kevin's music therapy sessions for several years and found the therapy a truly healing experience for me, too. Over time, we safely bonded through the music and related more comfortably to each other as two individuals, separate from our roles as mother and son. Kevin even began to call me Patricia after calling me Pat for eight years. I was shocked when he broke this pattern. Music therapy taught us healthy behaviors and helped us to let down our defenses. We experienced its soothing influence, which sparked in us a fun relationship of walking together, exploring restaurants, and laughing at our own special jokes.

As a part-time paid employee, Kevin has worked successfully under full supervision at three different companies. Presently, he is holding down a part-time volunteer job, working beside me at the public library. Kevin spends his other weekdays in a day center for persons with disabilities, where he participates in recreational classes and outings.

Working on specific tasks, such as unpacking books or sorting books, has helped Kevin use his eyes and hands to develop focus and stay grounded. He has learned to compose himself fairly well in public although he tends to let his inhibitions out at his day center. Mainstreaming in a work environment gives him exposure to good role-models.

At the present, when I accompany Kevin out in public, he has much better control over his aggressions than he used to. Since he is cheerfully distracted by strangers, I walk briskly beside him and grab his attention. However, every day with him is a new story with a twist of drama and humor.

His playful, trusting nature can invade others' boundaries. As a buffer between him and others, I often lighten up awkward situations by humoring him or excusing him to strangers. I literally stand in awe of other people's tolerance and compassion toward my son with Tourette syndrome.

Now twenty-nine years old, Kevin is still living in the group home with five other men under full staff supervision.

Having lived in his home for ten years, he is happy and comfortable. Though the group home has undergone many staff changes, living with the same guys for years has provided him stability and consistency.

Through twenty years, my son presented me many opportunities to empower myself. During Kevin's sudden rage attacks in social situations of our past, I experienced highly charged traumas that brought me shame and pain. I still carry faint memories of a young Kevin kicking me in front of strangers in public or an older Kevin wildly cursing at me in a restaurant or in a car. In spite of these unforgettable events, my hypervigilance has been dissipating through the years. For the most part, I have learned to rely on my own strength and emotional stamina. I confidently believe that I can endure rough spells with him, if I passionately sing to him, shock him with an off-the-wall comment, or just leave him alone. We still listen to Enya's music—a favorite from therapy—and take turns singing in the car.

When I reflect upon our journey together, having healed old wounds and dissolved ghosts from our past, I see him as a blessing in my life. Kevin, a gift from heaven, has given me the chance to practice calmness and to learn the art of loving.

3

~

Sudden Intruder

Babies are and have always been truly the most precious beings in the world to me! Even today, a few tears come to my eyes at the sight of an adoring mother holding her dear baby in her nurturing arms.

Since I was a young girl of thirteen, I've had recurring dreams of babies. The baby "dream" was powerfully rooted in my early childhood when my father, "a baby doctor," took me on his morning rounds to visit the newborn babies at his hospital. I delighted in naming the babies myself as I walked down the row looking through the nursery window, "Flopsy, Mopsy, and Cottontail." When I told Daddy I wanted to take one of the babies home with me, he said that I would have to wait until I was much older.

After Mother brought my younger sister home from the hospital, I immediately asked her, "Can she be my baby?!" At last, my wish came true at the age of eight when I became her full-time nanny. I enjoyed "playing mommy" with her and dressing her up like a doll.

As a young adult, I spent many quiet moments fantasizing about holding a tiny newborn baby in my arms. In my heart, I knew that to be a mother and to have children would be the most fulfilling job I could ever have.

Two years before Kevin was born, I lived with an over-whelming fear of dying. During this emotional period, a gyne-cologist told me that I would have difficulty getting pregnant because of a hormonal imbalance. I felt that I would die if I didn't have the baby I had always dreamed of having.

During my first year of marriage, I felt insecure as a new bride. I endured a great deal of apprehension and gloom and even had a premonition of Kevin's disorder in the form of a dark cloud looming over me. In spite of my anxiety and de-pression, my spirits miraculously lifted the day I received the news of being pregnant with Kevin. My dream of having a baby was finally coming true! I felt honored and excited to be carrying a precious baby. Kevin rattled around inside me, giv-ing me a feeling of euphoria. In fact, in the last months of my pregnancy, I trekked through the Indiana snow in joyful an-ticipation of his birth!

To my delight, Kevin turned out to be a good, quiet baby, who enjoyed nursing at regular intervals. Truly a model baby and an excellent sleeper, he took regular naps every afternoon and always slept through the night. I felt blessed to have such an easy time with my adorable baby. He crawled for a long time before walking perfectly across the dining floor at his very first attempt!

At thirteen months, the dark cloud began to set in. Despite nursing four times a day, Kevin abruptly weaned himself from my breast, bringing me much grief and physical pain.

As a hyperactive three-year-old, Kevin got wound up around other kids at the park and knocked them down aim-lessly. His lack of empathy shocked me when I could see that he didn't feel any remorse after hurting the other children and making them cry. In dealing with his behavioral problem, I learned to isolate him from the kids and hold him until he calmed down.

How could my quiet baby have turned into such a rowdy child? I was truly baffled, but I convinced myself that he was just being a typical boy. Regardless, I found myself on duty all of his waking hours.

Having rocked Kevin to sleep as a baby, I continued my pattern of holding him whenever he was agitated or fidgety. I also held his newborn sister Megan in my arms and at the same time protected her from her rambunctious three-year-old brother. To avoid disruption from Kevin, I usually nursed my baby girl in a standing position. Dodging Kevin while nursing a congested baby required all of my focus and patience. Unfortunately, Megan was born with congestion in her ears, eyes, and nose due to allergies. Since she had difficulty breathing, she nursed frequently and erratically in short snatches, just the opposite pattern from Kevin's regularity as a baby.

For relief as a weary young mother, I discovered that a soothing activity for Kevin was playing in his sandbox. Under the hot sun, he shoveled sand into his plastic buckets for long hours. His sandbox gave him a sense of security, just as his playpen had.

Over time, I learned that a fixed routine provided structure for Kevin. Our daily schedule was very organized and centered around meals. He loved to eat anything, from fresh homemade bread to salads and vegetables. Cooking for my boy was fun and enjoyable. I pureed his vegetables and minced his meats in his little baby food grinder. What an easy child to please in the kitchen!

Although Kevin was over-stimulated by other children, he was generally a cooperative boy and helpful around the house. His handsome appearance and athletic body made him so appealing to me that I didn't mind dealing with his occasional impulsive quirks.

Because of his language delay, Kevin couldn't connect words until three and spoke in choppy sentences until six. However, he was not afraid of talking and showed no tension in his jaw. Though he had adequate hearing for language learning, Kevin's speech was hesitant in nature, and he used *well* and *um* for starters when searching for words and basic sentence structure.

As a five-year-old, Kevin baffled his father and me by waking up in the middle of the night terror-stricken. He was inconsolable! Disoriented, he sat up in bed and screamed hysterically with a frightened expression on his face. He was breathing heavily and sweating profusely. After fifteen minutes he relaxed and fell back to sleep, unable to remember the trauma the following morning. Shocked and distraught over his sleep problem, I had trouble going back to sleep. Fortunately, his night terrors did not occur often.

For two years Kevin had been attending a reputable Montessori school. One day his teacher noticed that Kevin didn't hear him when he addressed the whole classroom from the front. Since the teacher had a usual habit of whispering to his children beside their desks, Kevin's developing hearing problem had escaped notice.

After being notified of his poor hearing, I quickly rushed Kevin to a special hearing center, where he was diagnosed with a 40% hearing loss. A few days later, his doctor discovered ear infections in both ears. Since Kevin had never complained about any pain, I was shocked!

Antibiotics slowly cleared his ear infections. Soon after testing, an ear, nose, and throat physician recommended allergy shots. Because Kevin was allergic to his own bacteria, I gave him weekly antigens myself for four years. As a result, his allergy problem cleared up.

Around his sixth birthday, Kevin began to show signs of bizarre physical tics. I had no idea what was happening to my boy. *What was causing his weird grimaces? Why were his eyes blinking rapidly and his mouth pouching out? Why did he lean his head over his left shoulder?* And worst of all, *why didn't my son have control over his movements?*

I panicked, *Oh, no! Is my boy turning into a monster?* I was horrified, scared, and embarrassed, all at the same time. The other children at school noticed Kevin's strange grimaces and mimicked him. His new condition suddenly became an intrusion into my precious family, already feeling vulnerable in a new home in a new city.

In addition to his baffling condition, Kevin's language delay greatly concerned his father and me, especially since we knew he had difficulty reading. Because of his hesitancy and lack of fluency, he avoided speaking by gesturing frequently. He also cluttered multi-syllabic words and omitted stressed syllables. Being an English teacher, I naturally wanted to help him speak more fluently but realized my limitations in supporting him. What a frustration for my son to struggle with words while his younger sister chattered away so effortlessly!

During Kevin's second year in kindergarten, a well-known German speech pathologist tested Kevin. In light of his scores on the Wechsler Intelligence Score for Children, the speech pathologist documented that the twenty-point difference between his verbal and performance IQs indicated a clinically observed language disability. His central language was so poorly developed that he could not classify similar words into categories and, as a result, made his lowest test scores on *similarities.*

According to her observation, the left side of Kevin's face was not as active as the right side. He wrote with his left hand and turned his head to the right when sighting with his left eye. She described him as a handsome, cooperative boy, who related well to people and expressed a strong desire to talk. In her report, she noted that Kevin occasionally lost his train of thought and talked irrelevantly. When he was asked, "Why do we have to put stamps on letters?" he answered, "They might say 'Dear Kevin.'" She recommended that he receive immediate individual and concentrated language therapy from a skilled clinician who was both a speech and language therapist. She also recommended that the therapist type the sentences Kevin created and permit him to read them back. In addition, Kevin should be encouraged to talk simultaneously as he gestured, wrote, or drew with his left hand.

Following Kevin's evaluation, I felt that it was imperative for me to take him to her speech clinic. Even though it was located at a university forty-five minutes away, I justified the driving distance because I believed that the speech experts would facilitate my son's language development.

I am indebted to the speech pathologist for her medical observation of Kevin and her ability to identify his ticking, blinking, and movements as Tourette syndrome. She was the first professional to inform us of his disorder. Three months later, Kevin's knowledgeable pediatrician confirmed her diagnosis. He was fortunately aware of the drug Haloperidol (Haldol), an agent known to influence neurotransmission and provide relief for Tourette syndrome patients. While taking this drug, Kevin showed considerable signs of improvement. Reducing his tics, the medication curbed the involuntary movements in his mouth and neck but failed to control his eye-blinking. It also facilitated his completing sentences with greater fluency. I tolerated its side effects of drowsiness and yawning, but on some days, I couldn't bear his incessant eye-blinking and erratic behaviors. All and all, I was grateful that his facial grimaces and neck twitches had disappeared and that he could finally talk without too much tension.

Once again, my son's physical appearance was restored to a normal-looking boy. However, Kevin's emotional issues began to surface through school. His first grade teacher reported that he became upset easily, often yelled out, and handled failure poorly. His yelling reflected "difficulty in keeping a lid on his *id* as a Tourette child." She also stated that Kevin didn't respond in the usual way to classroom management techniques. For example, when his classmates voted to remove his name from the Good Citizens list as a result of inappropriate behavior, he reacted ambivalently, first by telling the teacher he didn't want his name on the list and later by saying the opposite.

A school psychologist observed that praise, encouragement, and time-outs had little effect in modifying Kevin's behavior. While testing him, she reported that he was cooperative, though not particularly enthusiastic. She described him as a handsome, brown-eyed boy with an occasional frown and a worried expression on his face. He never returned her smile and smirked once when arranging a sequence of pictures that showed a dog stealing a chicken. Though he made good eye contact while interacting, he looked preoccupied at other times, staring at his desk and making occasional sucking noises.

Although Kevin's language steadily improved at the speech clinic, he made the same scores on his second Wechsler test as the previous year, with his highest score in block design. According to the examiner, his Human Figure Drawing suggested aspects of helplessness. Kevin demonstrated to us his poor test-taking ability; his low verbal and high performance scores became a pattern in future testing.

4

Separation Anxiety

Kevin's father and I divorced several months after the onset of his Tourette syndrome. During the marriage, we had managed to spend some time communicating with each other while taking care of the children. We had shared an equal interest in them and their health. However, I believe our general anxiety about Kevin and his recent diagnosis of Tourette syndrome had affected our personal life and prevented us from focusing on our own troubled relationship.

When a psychiatrist recommended that my seven-year-old boy sleep in the same house every night, I began my journey as a single mother of a child with Tourette syndrome. Fortunately, I didn't have to deal with two children on a full-time basis, as Megan continued to spend two weekends a month with her father.

Juggling a busy schedule between teaching and being a mom, I drove Kevin out-of-town to a university speech clinic for language therapy four afternoons a week. Though his speaking fluency improved, his emotional behavior grew worse. Ultimately, the speech clinic could not cope with him, as his unpredictable temper tantrums became too unmanageable for his therapists. My greatest disappointment came the day Kevin was asked to leave. I was devastated, knowing that my son needed continual help, yet despaired as to who would support him. Truthfully, I found no other possible options at that time for his language therapy.

I was happy that Kevin had a caring relationship with his sister Megan. They loved to run and climb in the park and dress up together for Halloween. Since they were buddies and good friends, they thrived on their picture being taken (e.g., p. 56). My son was tender with his sister and spent many fun days with her. She, in turn, delighted in entertaining him with her animated puppet shows.

As Kevin approached nine, my daughter's safety became a much greater concern to me. I felt the need to be on guard because of his eradicate behavior, even though he had never struck Megan. One sunny afternoon on his ninth birthday, I got a wake-up call.

Celebrating Kevin's birthday in the neighborhood park had been a tradition of ours for several years. The park, which was a safer environment than home or the pool, provided a place where the kids could run about and let off steam. As a single person, I found this year's birthday quite an engineering project. While supervising the party in the midst of Kevin's hyperactivity, I served lunch and cake to a bunch of hungry, rambunctious children. Later, when I was clearing off the dirty plates from the picnic table, I heard a child scream from the top of the jungle gym. It was Megan sobbing hysterically and holding her forehead with both hands. She blurted out that Kevin had banged her head against the pole of the gym. Her forehead was bruised, and she looked distressed. I was stunned that Kevin had actually turned on her and harmed her. I couldn't bear the pain of this violent act upon his little sister who trusted him so much. The incident literally broke my heart so much that I blocked the painful memory until Megan recently reminded me of this trauma.

For the following year, I organized a safer birthday party on a round-trip train ride to a small town forty miles away. I was thrilled to create a more controlled environment for Kevin's birthday party, which was exciting yet safe for little boys! While supervising six boys and a girl roaming the box car, I managed to direct their attention through the windows at the waving hands and scenic views. It was a fun, successful celebration! Fortunately nobody got hurt that year, and Megan healed from the park trauma, despite her brother's increasing restlessness and unpredictability.

When Kevin began receiving pink slips at school because of his verbal and physical aggression, I became more alerted to his hyperactivity and inability to focus on his lessons. In spite of the school's emphasis on gifted children, Kevin's third grade classroom was a chaotic mess of hyperactive boys running around and bumping into each other. My son was a far cry from the gifted child that the principal was advocating for. Since the elementary school did not provide a special education classroom for children with behavioral problems, his principal called me frequently to pick him up for disrupting class. Regretfully, Kevin delighted in getting negative attention in the school office, where his inappropriate behaviors were being reinforced.

After Kevin's principal had called me several times at the university to pick him up, I surmised that she didn't want to deal with him. Yet, I made certain to finish teaching my class before I zoomed over to "rescue" him from her office. Following a decision made in an Admission, Review, and Dismissal (ARD) meeting to remove him from her school, he was quickly transferred to a school with a contained classroom for emotionally disturbed children.

On the home front, Kevin's hyperactivity made it difficult for him to cope with daily activities. He was obsessed with his clothes, often poking on his shoes or tugging on his socks. Furthermore, shopping with him for new clothes was challenging for me because of his ambivalence in picking them out. He changed his mind so rapidly that I became frustrated with him and nearly gave up on shopping.

When Kevin turned ten, his test scores indicated that his verbal IQ had decreased. Greatly alarmed by this fact, I consulted his psychiatrist, who feared the possibility of a brain tumor. Begrudgingly, I listened to the doctor's recommendation to place him in the state hospital while it administered a CAT scan and some other psychological tests. The hospital placement was the only avenue at that time through which my health insurance would cover extensive testing.

As a single parent, I realized that I could not afford to pay for testing on my own. Encouraged that my insurance would cover a thorough analysis by medical experts if he were admitted, I made the heart-wrenching decision for his short-term placement in the state hospital.

During his six months in a very restricted hospital setting, Kevin underwent major psychological changes. The first month he went into shock and became quiet and lifeless; all his affect disappeared. I was completely horrified that he had become such a zombie! Oh, how I regretted my decision! You can't imagine how this hurt my soul at such a deep level.

I was responsible for what was happening to Kevin! I blamed myself: *Why did I listen to the doctor and follow his advice? What was
the matter with me?*

When Kevin started hallucinating in the last few months
of his hospital stay, I went into shock. He obsessed that others, including me, were blowing air around his body. It was
during those moments when he got so upset and angry that
his rage attacks began. His obsessive-compulsive paranoia escalated into a physical confrontation that involved kicking me.
During my short weekly visits, I was anxious about respecting
his boundaries in order to prevent him from violating mine.
Although the CAT scan that the hospital administered did not
detect a brain tumor, Kevin was becoming progressively more
sensitive and emotionally distraught.

Not only was tolerating Kevin's changes a difficult experience for me but also interacting with his staff. I felt that they
discounted my knowledge of him and did not consider me an
equal team player, in spite of having known him all his life. I
perceived them as judging me a controlling mother and blaming me and his father for aggravating his Tourette's. Though I
truly wanted to receive their favor and respect, they intimidated
me. My daughter was scared at the hospital, too, and she didn't
even say a word during our family therapy sessions. I supposed
she was too anxious to share how much she missed Kevin.

Ironically, my son's condition had become more critical
several months after entering the hospital. I clearly wanted him
out of there! I was concerned that his behavior would escalate
even more if he stayed any longer in the institution. I also
wanted to experiment with another drug that the hospital was
unwilling to try. Against strong protests from his medical staff,

I boldly withdrew Kevin from the hospital and brought him to his old psychiatrist to monitor a different medication.

Kevin eagerly returned to my home, but he hallucinated frequently and became violent in my car. Still only ten, he angrily punched me in the stomach on the way to school most mornings. I vehemently urged the school bus service to pick my son up, but they refused to transport him to his remotely located school that was thirty minutes away from home. I had no choice but to tolerate his blows. Though Kevin's punches were not very forceful, they were stressful to me and extremely distracting during rush hour traffic.

Having to deal with his difficult behavior, I coped with the circumstances as best I could. When I tried putting him in the back seat, he took the seat belt off and put his arms around my neck. After that, I decided that the front seat was less dangerous than the back seat; yet, during severe fits of rage, I vividly remember stopping the car to pull him out onto the curb to calm him down. I learned that it was safer to handle him outside the car before his behavior escalated into intolerable blows.

His misbehavior in the mornings haunted me throughout the day while teaching. Though still hypervigilant, I recuperated in the safety of my own classroom, where I regained a sense of control within myself.

Megan endured a very disturbing period when her brother became hypersensitive to her breathing. Riding in the car, Kevin sometimes told her to stop breathing on his shoulders. As a young seven-year-old, she was startled by his sensitive responses. Unfortunately, she learned that her denials fueled his rage even more.

At this point, I became aware of Kevin's acute sensitivity to every movement, word, or action in his environment. Learning what his triggers were, I practiced being gentle and disengaged in any arguments with him. I made him take time-outs in his bedroom whenever the dark cloud of his rage attacks stormed in.

In his elementary school, Kevin's aggression toward other children was increasing in the classroom of his new special education teacher. He had frequent episodes of temper tantrums without any apparent reason. At times, he looked dissatisfied, unable to say what he wanted or to sustain interest in play activities. Regrettably, on the days when he behaved well at school, he misbehaved at home.

After a period of time, his explosive behavior began to drain me and wear me down. Our experiment with a different medication proved to be unsuccessful. My mornings and evenings with Kevin had become too emotionally taxing, even though he was responding well to an after-school care program. I was too traumatized and confined to my room. I had even hired a lady from a nursing service to help me out on the weekends, but she wasn't equipped to handle him either. On the day that Kevin threatened me with a kitchen knife in his hand, I got my own shocking wake-up call. In that moment, I realized he had turned into a violent, raging boy.

Weary and burned out on Thanksgiving Day, I resigned from my motherly duties by calling Kevin's father and asking him to take care of our son at his house. I didn't want to put his father on the spot, but I knew I couldn't survive another day with Kevin. When Dad bravely consented to taking care of him, a huge burden was lifted from my shoulders.

Kevin's violent behavior perpetuated during the holiday season. On Christmas Day at Dad's, my son destroyed the toys that he had hoped for all year. The day after Christmas, he had a temper tantrum in the middle of the mall, saying that others were blowing on him. Fortunately, his father managed to calm him down and get him in the car.

Two days after Christmas, I experienced a big disappointment. His father readmitted our disturbed son into the same hospital that I had fought to pull him out of four months earlier. After undergoing tremendous stress taking care of Kevin, he gave up. I didn't blame him for his decision, but I was saddened to find out that he was unable to manage Kevin any better than I had. These Christmas outbursts taught me another lesson about my son—Kevin had a serious condition that required assistance from a complete staff. As I was anxious about dealing with the medical staff again, I turned custody over to Kevin's father and proceeded to visit my son at the hospital on a regular basis.

While Kevin stayed several years in the state hospital, I participated in private counseling, which helped me to deal with the changes in my life. Fortunately, my counselor gave me guidance in interacting with the hospital staff.

I learned that the staff was just as confused about Kevin as I was. They experimented with changing his medication dose and also with placing him in a different psychiatric unit at the hospital. In accordance with their disciplinary procedure, they isolated him in a special bolted room for time-outs whenever he was extremely angry or defiant.

My restricted visits with Kevin at the hospital distressed me. I had only two hours on Sundays to sit with him in the hospital lobby. Since Kevin was not a talker, it was a boring set-up. Our non-private visits caused me to feel some separation anxiety because I was not really able to connect with him. My visitation rights improved the second year, when I was granted permission to take him out of the hospital on overnight "passes." Unfortunately, during one of his passes, a plumbing truck crashed into my car from behind. I learned later from his staff that he was really shook up from the accident on the following day.

In those difficult emotional years I managed to handle the challenges of the hospital system and my separation from Kevin. Because the staff felt that he needed to stay there longer, his father and I went to court to obtain an extension from the state. I will never forget the emotional trauma of testifying in court about my son's condition. I experienced great shame in describing the severity of his behavioral disability to warrant another year in the hospital.

Having little contact with Kevin, I lived with a disquieting feeling of not knowing what was going on. I had to give my confidence over to his staff and believe that he was treated well behind those iron doors. Hospital policy prohibited parents from entering the actual psychiatric unit, since strict boundaries were necessary to protect its patients.

I didn't learn new tools or techniques for dealing with Kevin's behavior. However, I had some contact with teachers in his hospital school, which was a part of our public school district. I appreciated its more relaxed atmosphere and their feedback about his behavior and learning.

During his long hospital stay, Kevin continued to show a steep decline in cognitive functioning. The staff reported his case as unusual, as a result of their inability to find any cause for his decline. My son's process in the hospital was extremely heartbreaking to me. I had hoped that his medical team would discover something significant about his condition.

Following his three years at the hospital, Kevin was placed in a residential youth center out-of-town. Ready for a less restrictive life-style, Kevin spent two very happy years living in a small dorm cottage with several other teenagers, enjoying outdoor games, swimming, and touch football. Freer and more relaxed, he blossomed there and chattered spontaneously, sometimes about nonsense. His racy mind rattled off names of rock stars and makes of cars. Listening to loud heavy metal music became his newly discovered interest. The repetitive beat and loud, elongated sounds stimulated and energized him. His obsession with the lyrics and drama of Kiss, Ozzy Osbourne, and Iron Maiden, as well as his fantasy to become a rock star, persisted for the next ten years.

My son's psychologist believed that heavy metal music was harmful to him. I didn't agree with the therapist but kept my opinion to myself. In fact, I wondered if music was the only pathway to Kevin. However, I never guessed that years later music would become his major form of therapy and that singing in his bedroom would be his favorite pastime.

At this point in my story, I find it important to mention that Kevin's interest in music was clearly rooted in his early childhood. His father, who was a pianist and a professor in the university music department, exposed the children to music at an early age and generously shared it with them in our home. Although they frequently heard classical music, Dad comically played musical interpretations of animals on the piano for their enjoyment. Because of the musical influences in Kevin's past, I wasn't at all surprised by his newfound interest in heavy metal music.

Strongly committed to my son's progress, I made the two-hour drive twice a month to see Kevin at the center and to participate in his therapy sessions, sometimes with his father. Unfortunately, our joint visit as a parent support team confused and disturbed Kevin. Seeing us together conflicted with his knowledge that we were no longer married and his desire for us to be together as his mother and father. We were utterly surprised at his awareness about us and his difficulty in accepting our long-standing divorce. Was his strong yearning to live with his father a divorce issue or was it a boy's natural desire to identify with his dad at age fifteen?

Since Kevin's physician at the youth center was experimenting with different dosages of Haldol, I decided to consult a doctor who was an authority on Tourette to determine his correct dosage. I flew with Kevin on a weekend trip to Memphis to visit the neurologist, then located at the university's Child Development Center. Having previously examined Kevin in our area when he was eight, the physician now described his Tourette symptoms as: "eye blinking, mouth twitching, especially on the right, mouth opening, tensing of his neck muscles with head movement, movement of his right chest wall and shoulder, and movements of various fingers and toes." He added that Kevin had some *palilalia* or "repeating of his own words" and recommended an appropriate drug dosage that was later implemented.

While living at the center, Kevin developed a new behavioral pattern, much to my chagrin. Acting on his impulses and following the leader of a group of boys, he trailed after them several times and ran away from his dorm cottage. Yet the gang wasn't too smart; each time they got caught.

During this period I got very alarmed at the risks my daring son was taking as a growing fifteen-year-old, even though he had run away before. His running away pattern took root at the center and later became the most prominent pattern in his life—his main outlet for expressing himself. Basically a loner with few interests, he kept his expression to himself. When his spirit wanted to run free like a bird, he found an escape from the humdrum of dorm life by bolting.

The head administrator of the center had originally planned to place Kevin in a large youth residential in a big city miles away from us. Taking my son's request into consideration, they, however, permitted Kevin to live with his father, who strongly consented to provide enough structure for him. Kevin would go to the local high school and also help his Dad at his delicatessen doing little jobs, such as washing dishes, clearing off tables, and mopping floors.

Our decision against transferring Kevin to a permanent youth residential was a turning point in his life. We were not ready to take such a big step. As parents we felt that we had not given Kevin enough support ourselves. During the last five years, we had taken a long break from parenthood while Kevin resided in the two institutions. We had missed him and felt we needed to resume more responsibility. However, his father was understandably concerned about his limitations in taking care of Kevin while running a new business.

5

Night and Day

As a fifteen-year-old teenager, Kevin fulfilled his dream of living with his father after his discharge from the youth center. He admired Dad and naturally wanted to please him. Sadly, Kevin's disorder changed drastically in nature during this trying period and escalated to recurring behavioral problems and persistent runaways from high school.

In the midst of his workday, Dad did his best to cope with Kevin's disturbing runaways. As the new owner of a deli, he underwent great stress in dealing with his business and being a father at the same time. As often as possible, he motivated Kevin to wash dirty dishes or help clear tables in the restaurant, but my son's defiance, inappropriate conduct, and runaways increased beyond his father's tolerance level. Even though Kevin was receiving psychological help from a state agency, he was still verbally and physically aggressive toward his father and his dog.

One day with a burst of newfound energy, I became inspired to take care of Kevin again, still only fifteen. Because of my regained strength and his father's distress, I convinced Dad to let me take our son on. Against the warnings of Kevin's new psychologist, I firmly held to my decision to let him live with me and my daughter at our house. Not giving up on motherhood, I wanted to allow Kevin another chance.

I was initially thrilled and excited to have Kevin in our home again; however, my enthusiasm soon wore off when the harsh reality of Kevin's inappropriate behavior set in. I was freaked out by his latest trick of climbing out of the second floor bedroom window and jumping down onto the patio. He frequently sneaked out of the house to run free through the surrounding neighborhoods or to scavenge convenience stores and malls for sodas. Megan was shocked to discover that her brother had stolen money from a secret envelope in her chest of drawers. After Kevin stole money from my wallet to buy sodas, I began to guard my purse by carrying it around the house on my shoulder.

Because of Kevin's compulsion for food, I put a combination lock on our refrigerator to monitor his food intake. Unbelievably, he figured out the code without damaging the refrigerator and raided the appliance. After this incident, I had to be on guard every minute, watching out for his compulsions and sneaky behavior. Feeling edgy, I became hypervigilant and conscious of Kevin's every move—a watchdog on duty night and day.

Whenever Kevin ran from my home, I learned to follow him in the car from a distance and not to chase after him. Sometimes I saw him running in the street instead of on the sidewalk. He ran much harder if he thought I was chasing him, and he refused to get into my car when I came up close behind him. One time I calmly asked a male stranger in a parked car on the street to tell Kevin to get inside my car. Under the third party's direction, he jumped right in. Paradoxically,

Kevin would get in my car if he was returning from the mall. At that point, he complied because he had already satisfied his impulse to run.

His Tourette disorder made him terribly groggy and difficult to wake up. One morning after he refused to get out of bed for school, I left him at home alone. Later I heard from a friend that she saw him running along the shoulder of the freeway on the way to school. I was shocked to learn how bold and adventuresome my son was. Though pleased that he wanted to go to school, I was clearly disturbed by his obliviousness to dangerous cars whizzing past him on the freeway.

In Kevin's public school, his special education classroom for emotionally disturbed teenagers consisted primarily of rough street guys, many of whom had been neglected and abused at home. Since Kevin was easily influenced by the guys, his school staff was worried that he was learning inappropriate behaviors from them. Eventually, his special education committee requested that he be placed in an emotionally disturbed classroom of a regular high school under the supervision of its highly regarded teacher. Although the teacher's classroom consisted of troubled boys, I was reassured that they were from nurturing families.

When I first learned that the school was only two blocks from my office, I was very excited. I remember thinking of how convenient it would be to drop Kevin off in the mornings near my office. The thought never occurred to me that the close proximity would make it more advantageous for Kevin to run away from school to my office. To my surprise, one day a policeman arrived at my office with my son. Kevin had told the man where to find me since he didn't tell the officer he had left school. If Kevin had only known how much police officers intimidated me! I freaked out and kept Kevin at my office for the rest of the day.

As my vagabond son's restless behavior progressed, Kevin roamed the halls of the school during various hours of the day. Disappointingly, I found out that his teacher was not able to provide a well-supervised environment and keep track of his activities. In fact, one day he escaped from the special education unit and created a stir in one of the regular classrooms by walking in. Kevin was making bold attempts to find his own niche in the school. What a determined guy!

Within a short period of time, Kevin's teacher grew impatient and was eager to get rid of her wandering student. Due to the difficulty involved in supervising him, Kevin was transferred to a high school for teenagers with special needs. At his new school, Kevin refused to identify with most of the students, who were either mentally retarded or physically impaired. What a challenge he had adjusting to an entire school for teenagers with disabilities after schooling with a group of troubled street boys! Unfortunately, Kevin never seemed to fit into any particular classroom.

His favorite classmate was a beautiful, high functioning girl named Maggie. Her warm smile, loving voice, and long brown hair lit Kevin up like a light bulb! Her soothing nature and gentle flirting brought him out of his shell. When Maggie's mother later withdrew her from school, Kevin and I mourned. Her presence has remained in his heart, and from time to time he has referred to her as his girlfriend.

Considered a loner, Kevin related better to teachers in his new school than he did to peers, except, of course, for Maggie.

My son was uniquely one of a kind and would have fallen between the cracks unnoticed if he hadn't been so dramatic in his behavior. And dramatic he was! Everyone in the school knew who Kevin was. He had a mind of his own and tested teachers and students right and left. If he wanted to do something, he would find a way to do it. For example, he might lay down on the floor during class or suddenly leave the classroom without permission.

Even though the emphasis in his high school was on vocational training, Kevin demonstrated a proficiency in a wide variety of sports and activities: bowling, basketball, basic conditioning exercises, baseball, track and field, jogging, and card games. Nevertheless, he complied with the school curriculum that specialized in training and preparing its students for employment opportunities on site.

Watering plants in the greenhouse and placing paper wrappers on hangers were some enjoyable activities that helped him acquire good manual dexterity. Though he was the best carrot chopper in the school kitchen, he proved to be uncooperative with the required clean-up. He also worked in the school's commercial laundry for four years. After loading and unloading machines, he folded towels meticulously and lined them up in stacks of twenties. In addition, Kevin got training in grocery shopping, preparing simple food items, and using city transportation. Generally, he received excellent life skills training, although we never trusted him to ride the bus by himself.

To further Kevin's intensive vocational studies, his teachers trained him at specific job sites. During his last three years he volunteered in the following community services or businesses:

a recycling center, the humane society, a church, a public library branch, and a motel. At the library, he cleaned records and changed "date due" slips in books. Kevin was able to do quality work when he focused on the task at hand. Although he was dismissed from the church and library sites within a month due to behavioral problems, he worked steadily for seven months at the motel. His pace was slow, but he always completed his tasks. Kevin meticulously cleaned motel rooms and methodically made beds. Then for eight months he worked once a week in the "Puppy Palace" at the Humane Society, stacking newspapers for the animal cages, but needed supervision to stay on task. Following this job, he worked daily at a recycling center on a variety of contracts.

Kevin's teacher, Ms. Robinson, worked very closely with him to provide the proper supervision and support during several years of high school. My son never left her side, and it was commonly known that Kevin was her pet student. They truly adored each other. He responded to her devotion and, needless to say, became enamored with her beautiful long blond hair. His high school obsession of long blond hair became rooted at this time in the image of his attractive and doting school teacher.

Her loyalty and dedication helped Kevin develop a strong imprint of relating to women one-on-one, and her female influence nurtured him and pepped him up. When she suddenly resigned from teaching a year before his graduation, he went into shock. Grieving her loss, Kevin was less motivated to concentrate on his vocational tasks. He lost focus and ran away more frequently to restaurants and service stations. The school became frustrated at his lack of compliance, and, though I was sorry about his behavior, I knew it was out of my hands. During a lengthy ARD meeting, his principal curtly remarked to me, "Kevin is the only student in our school that doesn't give to anybody." The reality of her strong words struck a chord inside me since I, too, felt hurt and wounded by his demanding nature.

In high school Kevin was capable of following directions and understanding most spoken words. Being a moody guy, his emotional state varied from day to day, and he was easily distracted. Whenever he was in certain moods, he wouldn't respond at all. He was known to withdraw from a situation and laugh to himself, showing disinterest in the happenings around him.

My son truly rejected his special school by constantly perseverating on attending a regular high school. (Perseveration, a symptom of Tourette syndrome and ADHD, is the constant repetition of a phrase, thought, action or question.) In Kevin's mind, he was unwilling to participate in a school that was not considered a "regular" high school for "normal" students, thus refusing to see himself as having special needs.

While observing his classroom one day, I painfully witnessed him crying and angrily shouting: "I want to leave this school. I hate this school! I'm not retarded!" He turned to me, and yelled, "Take me out of this place!" The principal rushed into the classroom to calm him down and take him to her office. I wanted to snatch him away and rescue him from his misery, but I didn't dare because I believed it was the only school in the system that would enroll him. This episode was one of the very few times in Kevin's life in which I actually saw him crying with tears in his eyes.

Wanting to deal with his demand to go to a regular school again, I decided to check out another school option. Kevin and I went to visit a special education classroom in a regular high school near his school. When I heard the phony, sing-song voice of the teacher, I felt deflated, knowing that this classroom wouldn't be the appropriate placement for him. By deciding against it, I realized that Kevin's speaking difficulties necessitated having a teacher who spoke in a natural tone of voice.

Since Kevin was quiet during the classroom visit, he took me by surprise when he obstinately refused to get into the car after arriving at the parking lot. Wrestling with him, I literally dragged and forced him feet first into my car. I wondered if his oppositional behavior was Kevin's way of taking his frustrations out on me with his current school situation. Exhausted and weary from the physical struggle, I cycled into emotional despair over Kevin's defiance and increasing anger toward me.

His neurologist experimented with the drug Orap for two years before we fell back on Haldol as the most beneficial aid to his Tourette disorder. Kevin's body responded well to its ingredients; in fact, it gave him the necessary support to finish high school and graduate at twenty-two. The sedative effects of Haldol slowed him down and reduced his runaways.

Although Haldol helped, I continued to seek other treatments. One day on a retreat, I met a chiropractor that had experience with Tourette patients. Since his office was in Albuquerque, Kevin and I flew there for a consultation. Based on a blood test, the chiropractor prescribed minerals, mega vitamins, and amino acids for him, starting at ninety-four capsules a day. Kevin needed cystine, phenylalanine, magnesium, B6, and others in large doses. I felt like a pharmacist popping forty-seven pills in Kevin's mouth both morning and night. Before I went to bed every night, I organized his pills for the following day. Over time, the number of vitamins was gradually reduced to fewer pills per day. I believed in the supplements and that they were helping him to get better. For many months he took them easily but, toward the end, began spitting the pills out, signaling to me that he was done with them. Poor guy, I didn't blame him!

As Kevin became healthier, he got more in touch with his emotions. As a result, he was becoming angrier, more violent and daring. Even though I was expending a lot of energy helping him, his conduct was getting worse. The good news was his repressed anger was coming out. The bad news, however, was his emotional outbursts were harder to deal with.

One night, after being hit and terrorized by Kevin inside my car, I stopped the car at a street corner near home and frantically got him out. Having a rage attack, he was wildly throwing punches at me. A male stranger at the scene advised me to drive home without Kevin, as it would be too dangerous to get him back in my car. Because my daughter and her best friend witnessed the trauma from the back seat, I felt humiliated and embarrassed for them. I wanted to save the situation with Megan's friend and, at the same time, deal with Kevin safely. Scared to death I would never see him again, I left my son alone on the street and slowly drove away down the big hill to our house. When Kevin came home thirty minutes later, I was greatly relieved to know that he could find his way home in the dark by himself.

His chiropractor gave me a booklet of spinal rehabilitation exercises for Kevin to do every day. He had recommended these specific exercises to correct Kevin's curvature of the spine and to strengthen weak muscles. At first, Kevin cooperated because of the newness of the activity but later was unwilling to exercise. The battle of coercing him to do exercises each day became too emotionally taxing and time-consuming.

After many seemingly long months, I became weary of the rigorous routine and emotional struggle with Kevin. My stamina was waning. During his fitful, angry spells, I was becoming more confined behind my locked bedroom door. It was utterly traumatic hearing the incessant pounding of his fist on my door, Saturday night after Sunday night. I lived in fear of the door falling in and having to defend myself face-to-face. So many nights I cowered in my bathroom, whispering on the phone to my girlfriend.

One unforgettable night, Kevin suddenly charged into my bathroom, raging and shouting obscenities at me at the top of his lungs. When he wouldn't leave my room, I was at my wit's end. He cursed loudly over my words, defiantly ignoring my firm voice. Though inwardly terrified, I maneuvered him into leaving by faking calmness. I knew if I showed any fear, it would egg him on.

In another incident, Kevin jumped on the phone downstairs while I was talking on the upstairs phone to a comforting friend. In both our ears he madly called me names and refused to get off the line.

Though emotionally drained, I did my very best to get plenty of sleep and to take good care of myself without the use of tranquilizers. Whenever I could, I took advantage of the few moments that I had alone to help me regroup. Yet, I continued to stretch my limits living in fear of Kevin's verbal and physical aggression. His verbal abuse had intensified, and his blaring jam box unnerved me.

Desperate for solutions, I invited a policeman to our home to give Kevin a straight talk about the consequences of domestic violence toward his mother. I seriously considered the idea of putting him in "the green house," a short-term jail for delinquent teenagers. However, the policeman warned me that my son would be exposed to negative behavior in the jail. Quickly deciding against that option, I became very frustrated at not being able to find the proper remedy for correcting Kevin's behavior. The man also reminded me of a key issue to my son's violent behavior: I was not physically strong enough to handle him when he was out of control, and Kevin knew it.

Lacking physical strength as a petite woman, I found myself at a disadvantage in the midst of Kevin's rage attacks. I had always perceived myself as physically weak in comparison to my older brother. During the present crisis with Kevin, I decided to take private aikido lessons to give me more confidence in myself and to learn techniques for gently throwing Kevin. Once, I even successfully defended myself from Kevin with a throwing technique I had learned! Aikido, along with lifting weights, helped me to feel psychologically stronger but did not provide a reliable defense against his rage attacks.

In spite of these traumatic experiences, my spiritual commitment to Kevin kept me hanging in there. Through my dedication I got stronger and began to believe that I was only given certain challenges in life that I could handle. As a result,

I was forever willing to endure the behavioral problems that Kevin presented to me. So I continued to give him vitamins, to keep my chin up, and to protect myself as much as possible from his rage attacks.

Eventually, I felt a stronger need to give more focused attention to my daughter Megan. I had been uneasy about her welfare from day one and, for that reason, had breastfed her a long time. Honoring Kevin's nutritional program, all of us abstained from eating red meat. Megan, though a young teenager, complied easily with the change in diet and enjoyed the healthy organic dishes that a lady cooked for us each week. But I knew I couldn't attend to Megan the way I wanted to unless I found an alternative home for Kevin.

In spite of his difficulties, Kevin had sweet moments with his sister Megan. One night while watching figure skating on television together, he asked if he could pick her up. She agreed, and he lifted her up in his arms in perfect imitation of the ice dancers.

Nevertheless, I became increasingly afraid that Kevin might suddenly hit or harm her, and I didn't want to press our luck. During the first two months of the summer, I had my daughter stay at a friend's house while I considered possible placements for Kevin. I brought dinner over to her every evening to keep in contact. When my friend said she was quiet as a mouse at her home, I hoped that she was not beginning to shut down emotionally.

Megan was three years younger and, while a head shorter than Kevin, had a strong and determined inner spirit. She demonstrated an amazing strength of willpower one day when she fearlessly pulled Kevin off my back. I still recall the power of her physical presence during that traumatic moment and her need to protect me from his sudden urge to hold me down. Megan was a role model of physical courage for me.

Fortunately, Kevin never targeted Megan, for he preferred to terrorize her cat instead by chasing him through the house. Cory was my daughter's prized possession, and she guarded him like a mountain lion. One day, Kevin picked up the cat with one hand and appeared to be on the verge of strangling him. Megan instinctively distracted Kevin by gesturing in his face. Cory swiftly loosened from Kevin's grip and outmaneuvered him by running into a closet and disappearing for several hours. Miraculously, Cory the cat remained undisturbed by his sudden outburst.

Kevin got progressively out of control during that crazy summer. Disregarding his sugar-free diet, he raided a local convenience store and devoured three candy bars. The sugar from the candy altered his chemistry considerably and set him into a tail spin that lasted for several weeks. At summer school he misbehaved by frequently leaving the classroom. At one point, he even hit me in front of his doctor during an office visit. Over time, Kevin's agitation culminated in the terrifying incident at my office where he threw me against the door and chased me down the street, thus precipitating his placement in a private hospital.

At this point, I regretted the decision that we had made a year and a half earlier when we turned down a transfer for Kevin to a private residential center for teenagers. We had not been quite ready to relinquish our responsibilities as his parents and had felt that we should give ourselves another chance. In hindsight, judging that decision was not fair, since we didn't have any idea how Kevin would behave living in our homes after his being away for five years. Both his father and I did our best to take care of Kevin and to meet his needs.

Placing Kevin in a hospital for the second time was a giant step for me. At this point, I was convinced that it was the correct measure to take for both our safety. I was making a more conscious choice this time, believing that I had done everything I could to help Kevin. My son was a handful, and I had reached my limit.

I also hoped that the therapeutic help at the hospital would assist Kevin in accepting the consequences of his inappropriate behavior and his personal violation of me. Since he wasn't aware of his anger and violent behavior, I believed he needed help in recognizing it.

I knew that I could not allow Kevin to ruin my life, which I felt was just beginning to crumble. I needed a life of my own and a chance to get my power back. Although my will was still strong, I was no longer a happy person.

6

Soda Man Running

After investing my heart and soul in taking care of Kevin, placing him in a private hospital brought me great feelings of loss. Though tender and vulnerable, I slowly began to recover from the painful experiences of that summer. As I grew out of my shell, I became motivated to create a new support group of family and friends.

During Kevin's hospital stay, I visited him at the adolescent psychiatric unit and also participated in meetings with his medical staff. According to them, Kevin perseverated on being independent and wanting to separate from me because "we didn't get along." I felt ashamed that he was talking to staff about our difficult relationship and refusing to participate in family therapy. Yet, I needed a break from him, so I was relieved to meet only with his staff.

The few times he saw me at the hospital, Kevin was as verbally abusive to me as he had been at home. On one occasion, he got close to me and looked like he was going to hit me. I wondered why he was feeling so angry toward me when I thought I was being a loving parent. I took it personally, *What had I done to deserve this abusive treatment?* I found it very painful to accept his aggressive behavior and his rejection of me at the same time. I didn't realize until later that he was not only being a Touretter but also a teenager. Kevin became a double dose of parental angst, and as a single parent I unluckily received most of the abuse.

Following two months in the hospital, Kevin's psychiatrist placed him in a residential treatment center for teenagers with behavioral problems. He continued his pattern of walking away from the center until one day he ran across town to my place. His brilliant sense of direction guided him home. Exhausted, panting, and drenched in sweat, Kevin shocked me and my out-of-town guest who had just arrived. I comforted my boy as best I could. Since his center was on the other side of town, I was terribly alarmed, *Was he really all right?* I checked him over, and he seemed fine. In utter disbelief of his finding the route home, I wondered, *How did he do it?* But in a second breath I gasped, *I hope he's not going to be running here again! What will I do with him if he does?*

A few minutes later, I nervously called the center to let them know that Kevin was at my house, since I supposed they were looking for him. "Yes, Kevin has been gone for two hours!" they exclaimed. The residence reported that his school teachers had sent him to the dorm to change into his PE clothes. However, he had bypassed the dorm and kept on walking. We realized that he must have been running the whole time. After that incident Kevin did not leave the premises again, as they watched him like hawks.

On weekdays the residential center transported him to the same special high school that he had attended while living with me. At this school they reinforced his positive behavior by giving him sodas, even though it was against my principles.

They thought that my nutritional program, which excluded beef and sugar, was too restrictive. The school and I differed in philosophy on how to take care of Kevin.

I was disappointed that Kevin didn't show any interest in making friends after school at the center nor did he enjoy interacting with his peers. He remained distant, self-absorbed, and detached from participating in various group activities. His verbal communications tended to be with staff on subjects that were extremely irrelevant or repetitive.

In their final evaluation, the treatment center stated that all of Kevin's behaviors were tolerable except for two: when he displayed aggression toward a peer and when he sunbathed inappropriately. Because of his wandering tendency and restlessness, they placed him on a close-watch program of escorting and supervising him while outside. Fortunately, Kevin responded well to their verbal directives.

Kevin's staff administered IQ tests and, on account of his low verbal test scores, officially labeled him *mentally retarded*. The new labeling enabled him to be an applicant for social security funding. At the same time, Kevin's father granted his custody rights back to me.

Once the insurance funds were close to running out, the treatment center gave me notice to find Kevin a new home. The center had committed to finding a placement for him in a MHMR residential facility. After their search efforts came up short, I frantically located a boarding home in a drug-infested part of town.

While visiting the only available apartment in the community, I was disgusted by the numerous cigarette stubs covering the entire carpet. The other clients were older men, who smoked and appeared to be over-sedated on prescription drugs. I cringed at the thought of kicking Kevin out of my nest into a wolves' den of older men's habits. I greatly feared Kevin would learn to smoke. I remember feeling such mental anguish and inner turmoil during my decision-making process. The only other option, which was just as unappealing, was having Kevin live with me. I opted for the boarding home rather than taking him in and being subjected to his behavioral problems. Holding my breath, I trusted that this placement was only a temporary measure for him and would lead to a more permanent home.

Suddenly my quiet life without Kevin was jolted into overdrive. Every day, the landlord kept me posted on Kevin's runaways. We assumed that he was scavenging the neighborhood stores for sodas. (Since soda pop was his main addiction, he never tried smoking, at least to my knowledge.) He stayed at that apartment for only a few months until the owner transferred him to the other boarding home operated by his wife, located safely outside of town.

His teachers and I agreed that this placement was more appropriate for Kevin. Because of its seclusion from town, we hoped that he would not run away. To our surprise, he persisted in running into town along winding country roads. Kevin targeted the same convenience store for sodas, and, unfortunately, his boarding home staff was rarely available to rescue him from town. Somehow he managed to find his way back home by himself. What a relief!

Kevin's passion at the boarding home was searching for sodas among fellow boarders. Was he really seeking stability in his life? Poor guy! During one year, he had lived in so many homes—five residences! Or was his urge for sodas merely a compulsion? One day Kevin literally received a whack on the side of his head! After stealing a soda from one of his fellow boarders, Kevin was fisted on the head by the man. My son was immediately rushed to the emergency room. Luckily, he seemed to be uninjured. I wondered at the time if the head blow was a karmic payback for the one he had given me at my office three years earlier.

Because the landlady of the boarding home had her hands full taking care of young children, I received little feedback from her about Kevin. At that time, I prayed a lot concerning my son's day-to-day mishaps. The woman did report to me that Kevin's lengthy showers were alarming to her and also were depleting all the well water. Also, his compulsive behavior of throwing his clothes away in her dumpster was getting out of control. He even tore up his clothes sometimes. All of these behaviors brought me anguish. When I was notified that he only had four pieces of clothing left, I bought his new clothes from a discount store, keeping in mind that they would eventually be thrown away. What a nature boy! I often thought that it would be cheaper for Kevin to run around in the nude, but he would be arrested for that, and I would be in deeper water!

Ultimately, I found an appropriate group home for Kevin, despite its location in a rough part of town. His speech pathologist, who had heard through school of the home's opening, knew of some other schoolmates who were interested in living there. I was extremely grateful to her for giving me the tip and pleased that he would be able to live with his friends in a home so close to school.

Soon after Kevin turned nineteen and moved into his group home, I was granted guardianship of my son by the court, declaring him incompetent in making good decisions. As his guardian, I hoped that Kevin would be able to adapt easily to his new home. At least, I felt assured that it was far enough away from my house to keep him from running here. Boy, was I wrong! Late one night he showed up in my carport just as I was driving in. Poor Kevin! He was dehydrated and drenched with sweat. After giving him gobs of water, I drove him home. Following this incident, I feared that he would run to my house again, but ironically he never did.

On account of Kevin's difficulty in adjusting to his new home, he developed a compulsive habit of phoning me incessantly on the weekends. He called me ten to fifteen times a week! He gave me the same line every time, demanding me to pick him up and take him "away from that place." Fortunately, I used his constant calling as an opportunity to overcome my guilty conscience by telling him "no" over and over again. Even though he was living away from me, I still felt that I had no life of my own. He continued to think of my home as his permanent residence and, in his heart, still wanted to live with me. While he eventually adapted to his friendly circumstances, he never completely accepted his new home; from time to time, he got homesick and perseverated, asking if he could move back in with me.

My son's most persistent misbehavior became his continually running away from his group home and high school. On occasion, Kevin sneaked out of the home for several hours during the night. Most of the time, the police and the group home staff couldn't find him; yet, one morning at three a.m., staff found him nude in the next-door neighbor's swimming pool. Several times Kevin even knocked on neighborhood doors innocently asking for sodas. He also walked into an unlocked home across the street, found a soda in the refrigerator, and brought it home. Eventually, I learned to accept his behavior and to trust he would return home safely on his own.

For a few years the group home staff gave Kevin sugar-free sodas as a reward for his good behavior in the group home and at the day workshop. Sodas aroused his interest and, to our knowledge, were his only positive reinforcer. Typically, he earned as many as five sodas a day and sneaked two to three more from his home's refrigerator. Over time, we learned that the more he drank sodas, the more he craved them. Unknowingly, we were feeding his addiction, and thus he was becoming more hyperactive and demanding.

His soda addiction caused tension among group home staff, particularly female staff. One unforgettable clash persisted between Kevin and a staff member. During that year, Kevin developed a love-hate relationship with Helen, a beautiful young girl of twenty who had the courage to work in a group home full of males. Unfortunately, Kevin became her major challenge; her long brown hair and sculpted fingernails were too stimulating for him. In fact, one day my son even grabbed a soda can out of her hand while she was drinking. The crowning blow happened the day he hit her on the head, seconds before I arrived to pick him up. After this incident and several other milder attacks, she finally left her post at the home. I felt terrible about Helen being targeted by Kevin, just as I had been in the past. However, I was relieved when she finally decided to move on and take care of herself.

When my son scared off a second female, who was his new manager, the director of his group home decided to hire a male staff member to control the aggression among the clients. Rodney, a nurturing, sensible family man, soon arrived on the chaotic scene as manager and quickly brought it under control.

During that same dramatic year, Kevin made nearly fifty unauthorized departures from his home. Staff would usually find him along the street nearby if they scouted for him immediately. He also escaped from school to find sodas at restaurants and stores. Since Kevin gave my phone number to service stations and restaurants, their frequent calls were disturbing to me. Whenever I was unavailable to pick him up, the police were called. I am grateful to those kindly men, who returned him home safely.

When I eventually refused to pick Kevin up, I told the police to call his group home and get their assistance. I did not want to reinforce Kevin's way of manipulating me by expecting me to rescue him. Yet, I was glad that he faithfully remembered my phone number, so I could serve as a relay person for him. For this reason, I have kept my phone number the same over the years to make myself available for my son, in case of an emergency.

Kevin's staff members and I didn't dare permit him to carry money on him, because we knew it would rapidly liquidate into sodas. Of course, having no money in his pocket didn't stop him; his friendly smile and big chocolate-brown eyes could easily charm generous shoppers into giving him nickels and dimes. Strangers felt sorry for him; shockingly, he turned into a charming little beggar. My proper upbringing couldn't handle it!

After my son stole a six-pack of sodas from a convenience store several times, I drove him there to have him give a direct apology to the manager. I also explained that I was responsible for Kevin as his guardian and that his disability had caused him to steal. Following that incident, I decided to show Kevin the consequences of breaking the law. If I didn't give him a stronger reality check, I was afraid that his stealing problem would worsen.

On a tour of the city jail, a sheriff friend of mine exposed Kevin to some inmates. Together with a friend, we saw scruffy men leaning against the bars at the front of a cell. My son was stunned by these real-life criminals—people that he had only seen on television. The sheriff led us into one of the cells to show him how confined it was. Kevin learned that the inmates lived at the jail, ate only sandwiches, and couldn't run off to restaurants for sodas. I firmly told him that these guys had broken the law and that he, too, had broken the law by stealing sodas. After that day, his stealing compulsion came to an abrupt halt. Thank goodness!

Kevin's staff and I believed that sugar and caffeine overstimulated him, altering his chemistry and stirring up inappropriate behaviors. All of us finally concluded that, by giving him sodas, we were encouraging him to run away to find them. I remember the scary day that we unanimously made a decision to discontinue giving him sodas for his positive behavior and to substitute juice, yogurt, or granola bars. We knew we needed to try something different to keep him safe, but we were scared and worried about how Kevin would react without his long-term soda reward. After we bravely prohibited Kevin from drinking them, he underwent a challenging adjustment period during withdrawal from his chemical dependency. We had certainly stirred up trouble for him!

In withdrawal, Kevin ran away several times during the day from his workshop to a neighboring grocery store. As a result, staff assigned a specific person to supervise him one-on-one in the workshop. Back at the group home, Kevin kept staff on their toes when they had to jump in the van and chase after him, the minute the door alarm went off. Once the buzzer sounded, his home was hopping, and even some of his housemates took part in the rescue team. Each time Kevin ran away, he had a funny smile on his face, since he enjoyed playing this control game and making staff chase madly after him. Boy, was he a real nuisance to his staff!

Kevin's running situation developed into an administrative focus, and his staff notified me to find another group home. They were afraid his running around in a drug-related neighborhood was too dangerous. I also believed that his behavior was too challenging for staff to deal with. At this time, I despaired while pursuing fruitless leads for another home.

After a few months of soda sobriety, Kevin's urge to run away diminished. Whenever he asked for sodas, they redirected him by having him do exercises in the group home, such as push ups, to work off his excessive energy. The exercise activity replaced the sodas and also helped to bring his chemistry into balance. Since his running activity had slowed down, the group home director informed me that he could continue living there. What a sigh of relief!

Kevin's soda fixation did not entirely go away, however. Whenever he wanted a soda, I sternly reminded him about his promise to drink water. I remember the day in a small restaurant when he tried to sneak over to the soda fountain. I shouted across the room to him, "Get back to your table!" Shocked by my boldness, Kevin surrendered to my command. I was surprised our spectacle didn't faze anybody.

By taking a stand in public against sodas, I empowered myself and overcame social embarrassment. In another incident Kevin hollered, "I hate this food!" when I didn't permit him to have a soda in an airport restaurant. I bravely responded by giving a public apology to the startled customers. In such a tense moment, I found the people to be very forgiving.

At one of Kevin's jobs, he harassed employees almost daily for sodas and sneakily rooted for them in their sack lunches. Just being around soda machines got his adrenaline flowing and totally distracted him from his own lunch.

While working as a bus boy at a Mexican restaurant, Kevin sometimes cleaned up the tables by drinking the left-over sodas. Not even warm sodas turned him off. Little did he know that his sister Megan worked as an administrator for a bottling company. A humorous thought occurred to me that, if he worked for her, he would be too tantalized by the soda machines to get any job done.

Nowadays, Kevin occasionally asks for sodas, even though he knows what the answer will be. He easily accepts our refusal to give them to him. His unconscious mind is asking for sodas while his conscious mind is accepting water. I continue to be surprised every time he asks me, since the answer has been "no" for four years. Though sodas are a substance that Kevin's body remembers, I am able to redirect him instantly. Because of his brain chemistry and tendency to get dehydrated, I manage to have water bottles on hand for him.

Kevin's excessive need for water is symptomatic of Tourette syndrome. Since drinking water is beneficial for increasing focus and improving memory, Kevin is more centered after drinking it. He manages sufficient control over his intake, but, if he is really thirsty, he can guzzle a liter of water in a few minutes with the same gusto as a can of soda. In fact, I have trained his day center to give him water consistently. Everyone who works with him knows that water is his lifeline.

I hope and pray that Kevin's soda running days will soon be over! Recently, he got lost on a library tour with his class and was caught drinking a soda behind the locked door of a bathroom stall. Tricky soda man found the john a good hiding place! Because Kevin's thirst buds get triggered within 100 feet of a soda, we stay vigilant at all times. I must say, his playful soda game keeps us alive and running!

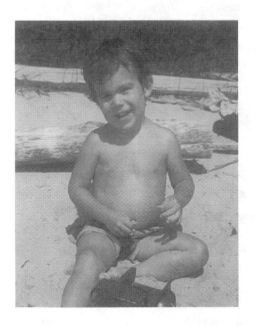

Young Kevin is soothed by the sandy beach and California sun.

When he's 3, Kevin enjoys playing ball and drinking apple juice at the park.

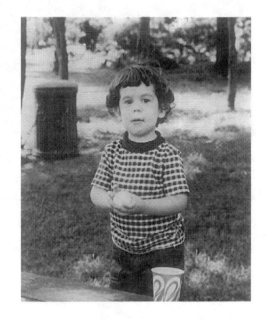

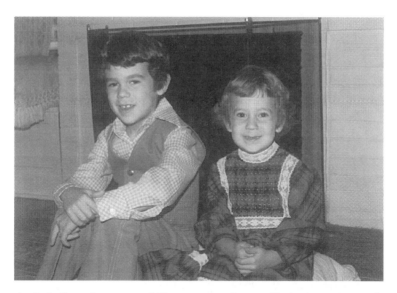

At 5, before the onset of Tourette syndrome, Kevin is posing with his playmate/sister Megan in his Austin home on Easter Sunday.

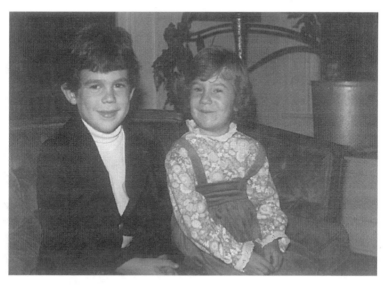

At 6 Kevin is diagnosed and put on Haldol to control facial grimaces and facilitate his speaking fluency.

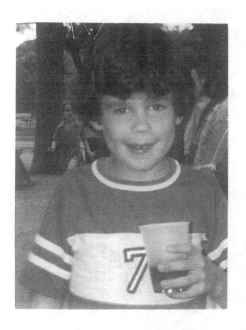

At 8 Kevin grins while drinking his favorite soda.

At 9 Kevin swims daily at local center working out his tics and hyperactivity.

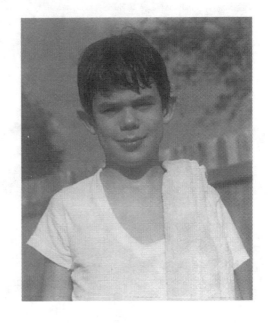

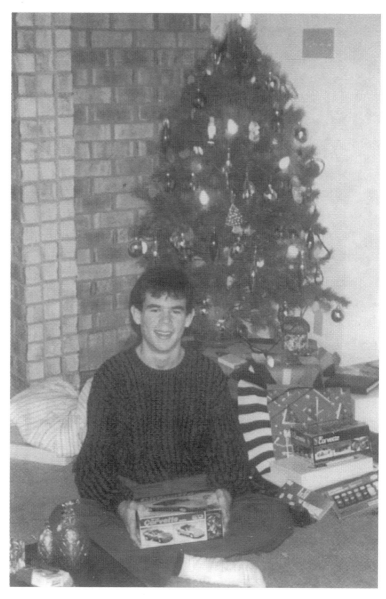

At 15 Kevin is happily spending his first Christmas home with his Dad after five years of living in state facilities.

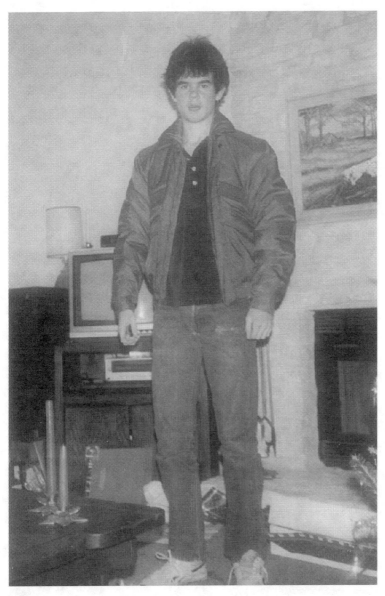

Restless and long-legged at 16, Kevin begins running away from home and later his treatment center.

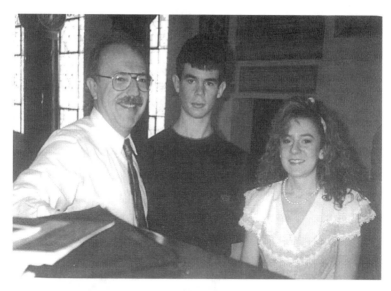

At 19 Kevin, accompanied by his sister Megan, enjoys hearing his Dad play the organ at his church.

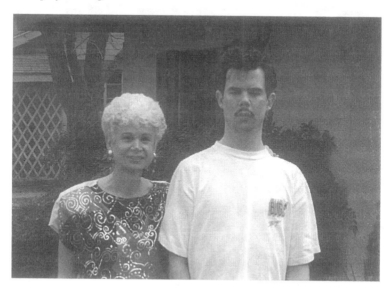

At 21 Kevin is overly sedated on Haldol. His doctor begins to taper his dosage while monitoring his TS symptoms.

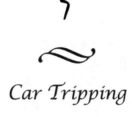

Car Tripping

I will never forget the traumatic events that happened as a result of Kevin's violent outbursts of rage at age twenty-two. I recall one of the most shocking experiences of all. We were driving in my immaculate new car on the freeway to another city a few hours away to visit a neurologist. Fixated on the oncoming traffic, Kevin started jabbering about the cars. Their flashing movement was freaking him out. Suddenly he was out of control and shouting obscenities in my ear with great intensity.

Instinctively I pulled over to the shoulder of the road. He banged his fist against the window. I was terrified that he would break the glass. He quickly grabbed my wrist. When he let go, I was startled by the blood on my arm. Kevin's long fingernails had ripped into his palm while hitting the window. He calmed down, but this moment was the eye of the storm. He madly began twirling his feet below the dashboard and then raised his kicks higher and higher. With a shattering crash, his feet smashed the windshield! *Oh, my precious car!* Completely stunned, I stared at the spider web formed on my windshield. I couldn't believe what was happening! Was this for real! And we were stranded out on a freeway in broad daylight! I wanted to panic, but I was in such shock that I remained cool and quiet.

Being in the moment, I jumped out of the car like a rabbit and ran to the other side. By this point, Kevin's fury had come to an end. I opened his door and pulled him out. Embracing him in my arms with motherly reassurance, I repeatedly told him, "You're safe here. You're okay." Limp and exhausted, he leaned against me and allowed me to hold him for several minutes until he calmed down completely.

While standing on the side of the freeway for only a few minutes, time froze as cars whizzed by us during this emotional moment. Unfortunately I still had an hour's drive to my mother's house, where we planned to spend the night. As I drove in shock, I prayed and prayed that he would stay in control. Every time I sensed his urge to explode, I stopped the car and got him out to help him stabilize. I had learned what worked, so I was willing to do whatever it took to keep us both safe.

After many scares Kevin and I finally arrived, all in one piece, at my mother's home. However, I chose to keep his accident a secret from her. My nervous mother would have worried herself sick about my driving back the next day. I managed to find some privacy to tell my sister about the trauma but hardly slept at all that night.

At our next morning's doctor appointment, I asked the neurologist to prescribe a sedative for Kevin for our return trip, but he told me pointblank that it was my responsibility to get him back. Wanting him to knock my son out with a magical pill, I was very disappointed not to receive any immediate help from the doctor.

The shattered windshield cast a gloomy spell on our trip home. Vigilant and determined, I completed the drive back. During our return at the same point where the accident had occurred the day before, Kevin started getting agitated again. I quickly took the initiative to pull over onto the shoulder of the road and take him out of the car. I wondered if the increasing number of oncoming cars speeding by was overly stimulating for him. Once again, I became aware of Kevin's sensitivity to movement.

Following the accident, I was in total shock for months afterwards. I had my car windshield promptly replaced to wipe out the memory of the trauma. I was numb for several days until I retraced with a friend that day's course of events. I realized that I felt extremely vulnerable and ashamed that it had happened to me in my car. My negative thought was that his behavior reflected some weakness in me that was unable to handle Kevin. I didn't want anybody to know about it, not even his staff!

Eventually, I disclosed the incident to Kevin's group home manager. He couldn't understand why I was crying, and just as I had feared, he was unable to empathize. At that point, I wished that I hadn't shared with him. He merely advised me not to travel out-of-town alone with Kevin in the future. Of course, his suggestion was a good idea, but I knew in reality that an accident could occur at anytime anywhere, even driving a short distance in my own city.

Even though I felt bad about the accident, I reassured myself that I was empowered through this experience; I had survived and was able to attend to Kevin in the midst of his rage and anxiety. Though my pride was hurt, I was unharmed physically and knew I would gradually recover from the emotional trauma. I had gained strength and proven to myself that I could stay on my feet during an emergency. I acknowledged myself for having the courage and stamina to maintain my equilibrium in the midst of sudden violence.

The car trauma was a reality check for me, letting me know that I was at risk anytime in the car with Kevin, but I discovered that I had excellent survival instincts and was a survivor through and through. The car episode did not stop me from driving in the car with Kevin. I still continue to drive him all over town and remember to sing to him if he perseverates or gets too agitated.

8

As Kevin's World Turns

During that same fateful year, Kevin's psychiatrist and I bravely decided to taper him off of Haldol. His previous doctor had prescribed a very high dose at 20 mg a day. Since he was overmedicated, the medical team and I wanted to give him a holiday from the drug. We slowly tapered him off of Haldol over nine months to observe his natural condition. His group home staff was curious about the real nature of his TS disorder, which had been covered up by medication for over sixteen years.

While tapering the dosage, Kevin became livelier and more affected. As his dose was reduced to only a few milligrams, he showed signs of tardive dyskinesia—a disorder caused by prolonged anti-psychotic drug treatment. We believed that this condition would dissipate over time, so we continued decreasing his dose to zero.

Two months after Kevin was drug-free, he was not functioning well. We were all shocked to see him in a highly nervous state. Overwhelmed by his anxiety, paranoia, and involuntary movements, he was unable to relax enough to eat or sleep. An emergency staff meeting was called at his home. His nurse was terrified that Kevin would have a psychotic break due to lack of sleep. He was agitated and hallucinating frequently, and his head was leaning over to the side in a strange posture. In addition, he was experiencing disturbed motor symptoms, making word tics, and eating poorly.

On occasion, staff observed Kevin running frantically out of the house. One evening, a frightening episode occurred when he darted out in front of busy traffic onto a major street near his home. Although he wasn't hurt, the police were called to the scene. Following this close call that night, the doctor prescribed a sleeping pill to calm him down, but it failed to lull him to sleep.

Worried and frightened for his safety, Kevin's staff agreed to place him in a respite care unit at a state facility on account of his explosive behavior and, in particular, his running out into the street. To help him sleep, Kevin was prescribed a low dose of Haldol to quell his bizarre motor movements and his agitation associated with tardive dyskinesia. Unfortunately, he endured another sleepless night.

In the midst of this emergency, I sought the medical advice of a specialist in neuropsychiatry, who regrettably was not available for new patients. Hand-delivering a letter to his office, I appealed to the doctor for an emergency consultation with Kevin. I reported that my son was in respite care because he hadn't slept for five nights and had refused to eat. I then alerted him to the fact that my six foot son's weight had fallen to 124 lbs.

When I arrived at the respite care unit that afternoon, Kevin was in an extremely agitated state. He suddenly grabbed both of my wrists and aggressively pulled me toward the heavy bolted door, demanding repetitively, "Take me from this place."

I struggled with Kevin as he pulled me closer and closer to the door. His hands gripped my wrists like handcuffs. I tried to maintain a calm exterior, but my frightened soul was leaking to the surface. Finally, he flung me against the door and demanded, "Take me from this place!" In my most subdued voice I responded, "You need to take your hands off of me." He complied just as the doctor appeared. I felt scared for Kevin and also helpless in front of respite care staff, as no one stepped in to help.

That same afternoon, the neuropsychiatrist consented to examine my son at the respite care unit, which was luckily close to his office. After talking to Kevin, the doctor immediately prescribed 5 mg of Haldol for his emergency relief. According to the medical doctor's observation, my son was markedly anxious and had difficulty maintaining eye contact, due to his gross motor tics. Kevin writhed with his head and upper body as he rapidly moved his little fingers on both of his hands.

Fortunately, Haldol helped Kevin to sleep again! After he returned to his home, his staff was relieved to find out they didn't have to watch out for Kevin's anxiety attacks that night. Having settled down emotionally, my son stabilized enough to undergo a complex EEG test, which the physician had recommended to detect subcortical dysfunction.

On the day of the crazy EEG testing, I was so nervous about going through the process with Kevin and about finding out more information about his brain. I will never forget that long afternoon. Upon arriving at the hospital lobby, Kevin showed his agitation when he shouted at the girl in the waiting room, "Orange girl!" She was wearing a bright orange shirt. I thought to myself, *How on earth is Kevin going to get through the test?*

To comply with the three-hour testing, Kevin had to remain still with metal pieces attached to his head in a dark room with blinking lights. Every time he jabbered, his body moved too much for the tester. I discovered that by holding him still with my arms around his legs, he was able to stay quiet. Whispering to him through the entire process, I reminded him of his reward of a healthy soda after finishing, if he remained still.

Praying in silence, I asked that Kevin would finish the test and that we would find out the necessary information for a clearer diagnosis. When he succeeded in completing the test, I was greatly relieved from the tension of crouching for several hours in the same position. The EEG did indeed validate that Kevin had a subcortical dysfunction in his left temporal lobe.

For the next five months, Kevin, his staff, and I endured the most challenging period in his life. The neuropsychiatrist had prescribed a second drug called Tegretal that precipitated an adverse effect on his behavior. However, we were slow to realize that the medication was contributing to his aggression and extreme violence. In addition, Kevin began to lose the six pounds that he had recently gained, due to nausea and a weak appetite. He often spit his food up or threw it away. Was his nausea a side effect of the drug? Sadly, he wasn't able to tell us.

As the drug dosage increased, unfortunately so did all three of his target behaviors: emotional outbursts, verbal aggression, and physical aggression. The latter behavior, which had never been a significant problem, began occurring two to three times a week with increasing intensity. Kevin's physical aggression precipitated various inappropriate events: throwing his TV out the window, kicking slats off the door, kicking a hole in the wall, threatening staff, running and yelling obscenities up the movie theater aisle, and blatantly spitting out his medication. He also shoved staff and engaged in violent cursing, stealing food, and frequent screaming. During the five intense months of drug trial, staff patiently coped with Kevin's runaways to seek employment.

Taking his group home manager along with us, I drove out-of-town to visit Kevin's neurologist again. Our companion helped me to feel more secure in the car, even though Kevin frequently yelled in my ear and grabbed my wrist most of the way. He also cried out that the police were going to catch him. Could Kevin have been sensing my own fear of the police while I drove at breakneck speed? I felt that it was an emergency that called for shortening the driving time. The headlights of the oncoming traffic were flooding Kevin's brain and freaking him out, as his anxiety level heightened closer to our destination. Nevertheless, getting the important information about a new medication was well worth the explosive trip to the doctor's office.

Disregarding my son's wild behavior as a serious problem, Kevin's neuropsychiatrist was unwilling to stop giving him Tegretal and to start him on the drug the neurologist had recommended. Taking action with the support of his staff, I abruptly transferred Kevin to a psychiatrist, who, in turn, tapered him off the drug. In a few months Kevin began to settle back to normal. His new doctor was willing to follow the suggestion of Kevin's neurologist to experiment with a brand new drug, which he had recommended during our second treacherous out-of-town visit.

After fifteen years of consulting psychiatrists, neurologists, and other specialists from Albuquerque to Memphis, I was thrilled to discover a new medication for my son that our psychiatrist would prescribe. As a miracle in his life, the drug risperidone had a soothing effect on Kevin and curbed his emotional outbursts.

9

The Magic of Music Therapy

A year before experimenting with medication, Kevin, at twenty-two, appeared distant and lost in his own world. I had given up hope that he would ever open up and express himself, and thus fit into society. Being terribly discouraged, I believed that no professional could ever help or reach my son in his own narrow world.

One afternoon, I was surprised when I received a call from Kevin's group home director, who told me about a new form of therapy called music therapy. The director called me at a vulnerable time, as I was feeling extremely hopeless about having any safe interaction with Kevin. I was still recovering from the recent trauma of his kicking the windshield in my car on the freeway, as well as from other rage attacks.

Kevin's director was eager to find an intervention that could help Kevin with his outbursts and behavioral problems. He wondered if music therapy might be an indirect approach to reaching him, since he knew that Kevin loved listening to heavy metal music on his jam box. He told me that, if I were interested in pursuing it, I should contact the CCC Music Therapy Center, which was just established as the first privately owned music therapy center in the world.

The concept of music therapy sparked my interest. I imagined it would provide a therapist who was well-trained in understanding and working with the emotional and behavioral aspects of Kevin's disorder. The bottom line was I did not feel emotionally or physically safe around him. Though the two of us had been doing our best to communicate with each other, we needed a skilled mediator. Miraculously, I received a call from Hope Young, the Clinical Director and founder of CCC Music Therapy Center (now called The Center for Music Therapy). She arranged a time for an interview before we received music therapy services.

During her interview, I became hopeful that participating in the music therapy intervention would help me to overcome my fear and intimidation around Kevin. Hope assured me that my son would develop healthier boundaries to inhibit his overly energetic nature and that I would feel safer with him over time. It appeared to me that the therapy would be beneficial for both Kevin and me.

Two weeks following the interview, Hope confidently introduced us to music therapy. When she first observed Kevin's interactions with me, she took note of his inappropriate, bizarre statements that were interchanged with frequent demands to me. His statements were repetitive in nature and constantly changing. For example, he would say, "I'm not going to kill you, Mother," or "You're not my Mother." Examples of requests to me were: "I want to go to college. I don't like it at the workshop. I want a job. I want to go home with you, Mother." Hope also observed that Kevin stood within inches of my face in a stiff body posture and bent over me while I responded by moving away and saying, "OK," or

"I know," with flat affect. Her awareness of his demanding personality helped me to realize why I felt uncomfortable and intimidated around my son.

From the therapist's point of view, Kevin considered me the person with the power over his life and his main avenue to getting his needs met. She interpreted his aggression toward me as his way of having power over me. Therefore, she recommended that Kevin engage in structured social activities, such as dances, house projects, and outings, and also in staff and peer one-on-ones. After Kevin began to socialize more and to establish stronger staff relationships, he became less aggressive toward me.

The music therapy intervention established appropriate physical boundaries through relaxing body postures and maintained socially appropriate distance during our interactions. Since Kevin's major issue had been oppositional behavior, the therapy permitted him to have considerable control in all our sessions to play out his control games.

Session after session, Kevin and I were able to bond through a mirroring process of imitating each other's arm movements to the rhythm of music. Surprisingly, he was able to mirror perfectly my arm movements and Hope's as well. Both of us were impressed with his graceful, rhythmic, and steady movements and his ability to follow every detail.

If Kevin needed to be in charge for most of the session, we let him take the lead during the mirroring. In such case, we silently followed his gestures, tics, and facial expressions, even if he just sat in the chair with his legs and arms crossed. However, due to his inability to communicate with us when he was finished leading, we were sometimes unable to judge how long he wanted to be in control. If we took the lead from him prematurely, he would withdraw, so we learned to observe him carefully and respect his need for control.

I was proud that Kevin learned to be a good leader. His command became clear and easy to follow. By practicing leadership, he eventually learned he had the power to communicate his needs to us. To reinforce responsible behavior and compliance, Hope consistently praised him for his good leadership ability, as well as his willingness to follow directions. Over a period of time, he began to respond in a more straightforward manner, giving up his hedgy way of communicating. Also, his frequent pattern of saying, "I don't know," subsided, and his sense of humor increased.

Through playing rhythms and communicating together with musical instruments, Kevin and I developed a close relationship. Hope created an emotionally safe environment, which encouraged him to open up. At the beginning of each session, she asked him what he wanted to do. Being allowed to run the show, Kevin picked out instruments with ease. He always chose the leader and selected the activities for the session, such as playing the piano or paddle drums as a threesome. When playing the piano, he decided whether we would play all black keys or all whites keys and who would lead the rhythms. Most of the time, Kevin played a sequence, and Hope and I improvised to his lead.

Interacting with instruments also assisted Kevin and me to experience a variety of ways to work out anger and frustration. By beating drums or vigorously shaking tambourines, we worked out our aggression. We also pounded on the piano together or hit a birdie back and forth with heavy paddle-drums as hard as we could. On the nights when Kevin refused to do mirroring at the beginning of our session, we sometimes hit paddle-drums for twenty-five minutes to release bottled-up energy. Hitting them helped him work through his control issue until he shifted into a more peaceful, cooperative state.

With the therapeutic use of musical instruments, Kevin woke out of his foggy state, and his mind became more energized. He was able to discharge tension from his Tourette symptoms and relax his body. Kevin and I also let off steam square dancing to country music while gracefully moving in unison as partners.

Kevin's tics disappeared while he was shaking or striking instruments, making movements, producing sounds, or singing. However, when talking to him, he continued to have a prominent vocal tic of repeating "uh-huh." Because this tic interfered with our communication, I learned to distinguish between it and a true "uh-huh" response by having him confirm his response with a "yes."

To help Kevin in developing a vocabulary utilizing feeling statements, Hope took photographs of Kevin, me, and herself that conveyed different states of emotions. Then we mounted the pictures on construction paper and wrote the feeling word beside each one of them. Examples of feelings were *blissful, peaceful, tired, happy, sad, loving, joyful, angry, scared, mellow, exciting, funny, hopeful, strong,* and *sorry.*

At the beginning of each session, Kevin was asked to point to the photo that best described how he was feeling. In turn, I identified my own feeling, and so did Hope. From session to session, Kevin picked *loving* as his favorite feeling word. One day, after being asked how he felt, he volunteered that he felt *glorious* and *peaceful.* Hope had never taught him the word *glorious,* and amazingly his face conveyed the authenticity of this word. Kevin had retrieved a seldom used word from the past. Wow! After familiarizing himself with basic feeling words, he began to internalize feelings and display more appropriate expressions of affect.

Using music as a soothing, energizing aid benefited me as well, when I started to experience my passionate, empathic nature. Through breathing I discovered a center inside myself, where I could rest in the quiet space between my thoughts. In this place I became still and tranquil. Feeling loving and warmth in my body, I forgot about my concerns for Kevin. Later, during difficult interactions with him, I remembered to connect with my center through circular breathing and calmly respond to him.

An important aspect of music therapy for Kevin and me was his learning appropriate boundaries and my learning to set limits for him. Hope taught Kevin safe and unsafe actions by singing songs with her guitar. She also demonstrated both safe and unsafe behaviors in order to show him how to recognize the unsafe ones. As a result, he became more willing to cooperate with us in following our lead.

The therapy assisted Kevin in taking responsibility for his actions and in accepting the consequences of his choices. He learned to distinguish between healthy and unhealthy choices. As the therapist consistently acknowledged his appropriateness, he received good positive reinforcement.

Always knowing what he needed, Kevin had the ability to select the CD with the perfect music for the mood of the session. We took turns on the microphone interpreting the music with our own unique vocalizations. To my surprise, I discovered him to be a great mimic. He imitated my facial expressions and my silly, animated vocal interpretations of the music while I learned to model and imitate his. Most of the time, his vocalizations were similar in pitch and range. However, one day he had a breakthrough when he produced a new high-pitched tenor sound.

To provide a relaxing exercise for Kevin and me each session, Hope guided us through a visual imagery. She noticed that Kevin rarely closed his eyes. In one guided imagery, she talked about loving yourself and saw his eyes begin to tear up. She realized that he had an issue with self-love, so she talked to him about loving himself. His body became so calm that he didn't make any tics for twenty-five minutes. Being in his heart, he looked so soft and gentle that he seemed hypnotized. I myself used the process as an opportunity to cry quietly and release withheld feelings from my past traumas with him. Afterwards, while driving him back to his group home, I remember experiencing a peaceful silence in Kevin that I had never felt before.

Nurturing each other became one of the goals for our sessions. Sometimes we reversed our roles, and I received a hand massage from Kevin. He followed Hope's instructions for the massage easily and enjoyed having safe physical contact. Moved by his ability to give nurturing touches, I experienced tangibly for the first time the power of receiving love from him. Within these tender moments, I teared up, and the harsh memories of our past began to dissolve.

Another nurturing activity for Kevin, Hope, and me was gently resting our hand on each other's palm while making circular body movements to the music of Enya. Because the movement had a hypnotic effect, we enjoyed doing it for a long time. Sometimes Kevin giggled and smiled while looking back and forth between the two of us and then laughed until his eyes watered. His face and mouth were relaxed. His energy was open, and he looked natural and joyful. During this favorite activity, we were able to connect heart to heart and feel a sense of oneness.

Role-playing served as a helpful activity for Kevin to learn new insights and behaviors. Since he adamantly refused to put on his seatbelt one evening on the way to therapy, we role-played the dilemma during our therapy session. In the game we both got in the pretend car and put on our imaginary seatbelts. Hope created a sudden crash in the car to wake Kevin up, and it was so realistic that I cried. She asked him to read the expression on my face, and he said that I looked sad. He seemed very alert and responsive to my feelings. Then Hope validated me by telling Kevin that I was a good mother to him and that I stayed with him no matter what happened. She expressed that he felt free to do whatever he wanted around me, since he knew I would not leave him and would always love him.

Following the role-playing session, Kevin again refused to put on his seatbelt in the car. Humorously, he fastened it later while riding on the freeway in the midst of zooming traffic. On some level he had grasped the importance of the safety issue. I was grateful that I was learning to give control over to him and to trust him to comply in his own timing. When Kevin finally fastened the seatbelt, I strongly praised him for making a healthy choice.

The Magic of Music Therapy

My most treasured session was the wonderful night our therapist videotaped Kevin and me interacting with the music. The tape captured Kevin's essence while he was in a relaxed state, even though he was a little shy in front of the camera. Although he had demonstrated many vocal tics at the beginning of the session, they subsided when he moved his arms or responded to my words and movements. I played the leader through the entire taping and extended my hands to encourage him to take mine. Sometimes he followed my movements and sometimes he didn't, but he continued to maintain eye contact during most of the time. Whenever Kevin disengaged or looked down, I drew him back in by talking to him in the rhythm of the music about topics of interest. I shared my love for him and my desire to help him find a job. On the tape I witnessed how powerfully we had bonded and recognized how emotionally involved he was with me.

Every session with Kevin was uniquely different but always therapeutic and educational, on account of his improvisations and the therapist's creativity. In one fun activity, we made emotive vocal interpretations to music over the microphone, based on expressive faces on flash cards. Kevin had fun imitating my silly vocalizations, and he giggled and smiled at my off-the-wall animation. Over time, his vocalizations began to vary and become more spontaneous.

We enjoyed a creative music therapy game called "red light, green light." Holding up "green" indicated moving or talking and "red" meant stopping the action. The player in charge of holding up signs would pick another player to do an expressive activity of either moving to the music or talking. Whenever Kevin picked me, he commonly held up "green" and asked me to move my arms. Because of his obsessive-compulsive disorder, he persisted in making me "go" on "green" for a long time, without giving me a "red" break. I continued to be responsive to his direction until I finally had to stop moving because I was worn out and realized he couldn't perceive my weariness.

When it was my turn to be in charge of the game, I held up "green" and told Kevin to perform a specific activity. For example, I would ask him to move his arms like a bird or act like a soldier. Kevin respected my command and followed my continued requests, such as moving like an Indian warrior or a dancer full of life. One day he shocked us with his accurate impression of a tough guy. Since I had no idea of his ability to make interpretative movements, I was astounded by his realistic impressions. In spite of his lack of affect in ordinary life, he was able to dramatize affect.

In some sessions Kevin was unwilling to engage in therapy. When he refused to participate, he withdrew in his chair by dropping his head and holding his body motionless. At first, we mirrored in silence every gesture, tic, and movement to connect with him and let him be in control. After a while, the mirroring process helped him begin re-engaging in the session and enabled him to give control over to the therapist. This approach was usually effective, but, on occasion, it wasn't. In such cases, the therapist and I didn't talk to him, for fear we might reinforce his behavior. We told him we didn't feel emotionally safe and moved to the other side of the room. Eventually, he came over to our side to talk.

During one session, however, Kevin isolated himself in the bathroom. I vividly remember our continuing music therapy for forty-five minutes without him. I even wondered if we should go home in the middle of the session, but I realized that Kevin was learning to make choices and accept the consequences. Because I wasn't willing to reinforce his anti-social behavior by going home, I let my son know my choice to continue music therapy without him. He eventually came out and joined us at the end. During another session, Kevin called me "devil" as we were closing. Since we didn't want to enforce this negative behavior, Hope and I left him alone in the client room and sang "goodnight" to each other in the waiting room without him.

As boundaries became the major focus in sessions, the therapist taught Kevin a self-defense technique after a housemate of his began a pattern of scratching my son's face. The therapist taught Kevin to protect himself from the occasional attacks by shielding his head with his arms crossed in front of his face and shouting, "Stop!" Practicing this technique trained him to defend himself from future attacks.

Just as Kevin confronted his housemate's anger, I had faced Kevin's angry side most of his life. Fortunately, in music therapy I began to see his gentler side and discovered that he liked to spend time with me in this safe environment. I realized that, as he mellowed through the influence of music, he had bonded with me. Ironically, Kevin began showing non-verbal signs of excluding the music therapist from our sessions. However, I felt that Kevin was weaning her so that he could just be with me. Hope also understood and gladly observed me facilitate the session with Kevin while watching and listening outside the glass doors. I really appreciated the value of leading the therapy in her absence. By this point, Kevin felt emotionally safe enough to let me guide him through activities that I knew he liked. He enjoyed my talks from the heart, as I told him how special he was. He thought I was funny when I became his outrageous entertainer. During our mirroring process, my animation motivated him to move his arms more freely and follow my movements.

Eventually, Kevin became energized by activities involving large motor movements. Marching proudly to the song, "Walk Like a Man," enabled Kevin to gain awareness of his pattern of stooping when talking to another person. After repeating this exercise several sessions, he stopped referring to himself as a boy. As a result, his favorite compulsive expression, "I'm a boy," changed to "I'm a man," or "I'm a dude." Kevin also enjoyed dancing to rock music and jitterbugging with a partner, helping him to focus and to relate.

As a music therapy objective, Kevin learned to identify his inappropriate staring behavior through verbal prompts and to correct himself independently by looking away. During the exercise the music therapist walked into the room, pretending it was a restaurant. When Kevin stared at her, she sang while strumming her guitar, "Look away, Kevin, look away!" Eventually he broke his gaze by turning his head away. In singing the phrase, she helped Kevin to ingrain "looking away" in his mind. Later, the therapist involved a third party to help simulate a real life incident. When Kevin began to stare at her, the therapist said, "One two, three, look away!" While some progress has been made in real life, Kevin is still learning to look away and to keep from giggling at people.

Realizing how visual Kevin was, his music therapist constructed a chart listing nine activities, from loud to quiet, from which he could choose. This format provided structure and a sense of continuity from one session to another. He could pick from the following: sing, walk, dance, skip, play drum, relaxation, play guitar, keyboard or xylophone, talk, or Kevin's pick. He commonly chose to participate in the large motor activities first, such as skipping and walking. Then he enjoyed singing and dancing to the CD of his choice.

Over time, we transferred our learning to real life situations. I set firm boundaries and began letting Kevin know when I felt unsafe with him in public. He complied with my limits and began lowering his voice in public after practicing voice modulation in therapy.

After role playing, "Excuse me," during many therapy sessions, Kevin was able to apply this expression to appropriate everyday situations. He has remembered to say these polite words to me at home or on the job site when he feels I am standing too close to him. In my perception, Kevin's ability to learn politeness has indicated a big step in his development.

Kevin's spirit woke up in the music therapy room and discovered itself beneath the mask of Tourette syndrome and medication. I had the blessing of witnessing Kevin in his natural state—relaxed and full of joy—without the interference of verbal and facial tics. Most of the time, he had settled into a peaceful state by the closing of each session. I was delighted to get to know his calm side. What a treat for me to see his true nature blossom!

Following years of music therapy, I noticed that he was more comfortable in responding to questions. As Kevin became more aware of his behavior, he learned to manage it more appropriately. And as he became better at self-adjusting his behavior, he was easier to redirect. Through the process Kevin calmed considerably, and I became peaceful within myself. I relaxed while slowing down to the rhythm of his dancing. Circular breathing facilitated our hearts to open and our bodies to relax. His loving eye contact showed a true desire to connect with us.

While participating in music therapy sessions, Kevin and I were able to heal on our past emotional traumas. As I learned to understand and guide him better, I became empowered. Although I was still intimidated by his disorder, I grew stronger and more secure around him under the music therapist's direction. I observed that Kevin released his feelings through laughter while I dealt with my feelings through crying. I also played the role of Kevin's tear gland, releasing through my tears his frustrations and pent-up anger.

During the three years of intense, interactive therapy, my son and I only saw each other during the sessions. Music had become the perfect tool that brought Kevin and me together to converse freely and interact safely with each other. By giving him choices to set stronger boundaries, I let him know what I thought was appropriate. His boundary development helped us to establish an emotionally and physically safer relationship. The therapy process had enabled Kevin to activate his right brain for better control over his body, emotions, and personal choices, in spite of his language disabilities. By moving and singing to music, both of us got more in touch with our hearts and emotions.

After undergoing traumas from time to time, I have participated in music therapy for my own healing, either in individual or joint sessions with my son. Though Kevin's world is primarily centered around his own needs, he can sometimes empathize with me during music therapy. However, one day he couldn't. I was upset and crying because of having lost my wallet the day before. His therapist asked him how I was feeling, and he answered, "happy." As tears rolled down my face, I realized that he was unable to relate to my unhappy feelings on that specific day.

Following this insightful session, I believed that Kevin needed more help in understanding his feelings and empathizing with others'. So I handmade and introduced some simple stick figures to his therapy sessions, whose expressive paper faces illustrate different emotions. Through these emotion props, Kevin is becoming familiar with his different moods. One day, he surprised his therapist by asking her if she wanted him to pick out one of the paper faces. Of course, she answered, "Yes!" After selecting *scary*, he dramatized three different versions of a *scary* face. His initiating communication with his therapist showed major improvement in his willingness to engage in an activity.

Kevin continues today to have his individual music therapy sessions once a week for an hour. Within the sessions he empowers himself through singing and playing different instruments. Though initially shy about performing, Kevin has opened up and now sings freely without prompting. He shows increased affect, especially during and after dancing, which seems to be his favorite activity at the moment. Occasionally, he chooses to take the session outside of the therapy room to the back yard. Lately, during his stimulating sessions, Kevin has been volunteering information readily and has become much more participatory and relaxed.

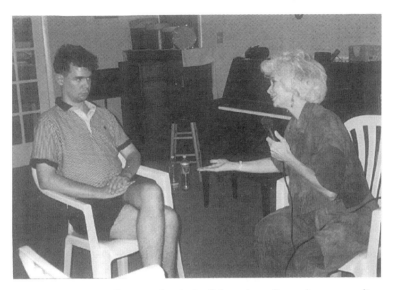

I am encouraging Kevin, who is in "shut down" mode, to vocalize on the microphone during music therapy in 1996.

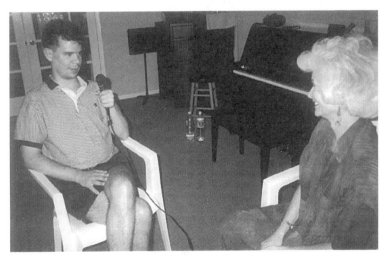

I'm letting Kevin be in control while patiently waiting for him to take his turn on the microphone in music therapy.

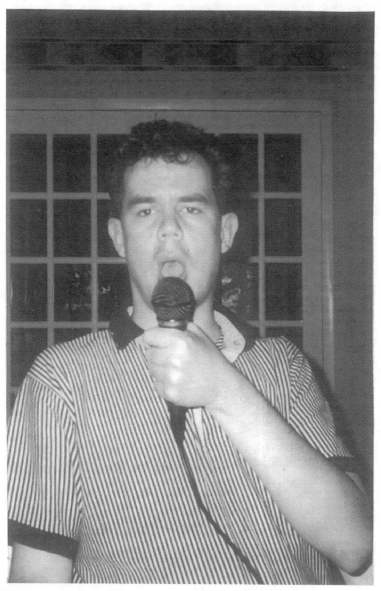

Kevin initiates performing on the microphone in music therapy. His vocalizations have improved his language and affect.

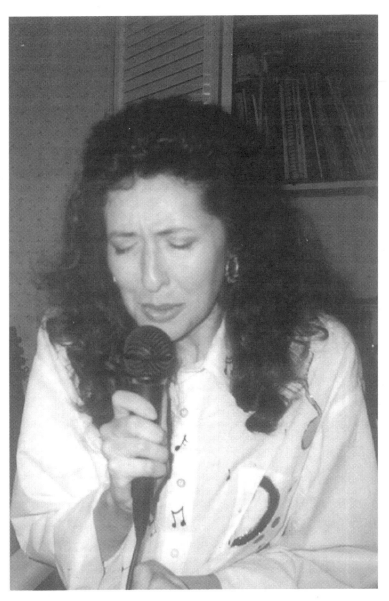

Hope Young, our music therapist, emotes on the microphone during a session to demonstrate affect for Kevin.

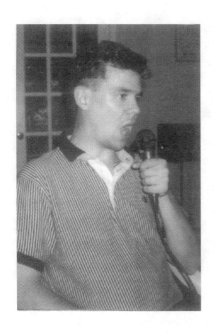

Kevin
vocalizes,
"Ahh."

I vocalize
back, "Eee."

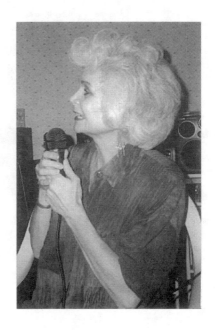

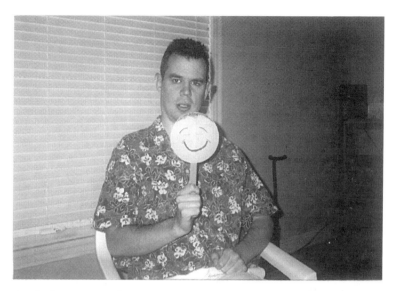

At the beginning of a session in 2000, Kevin selects *peaceful* from the emotion props to identify how he feels.

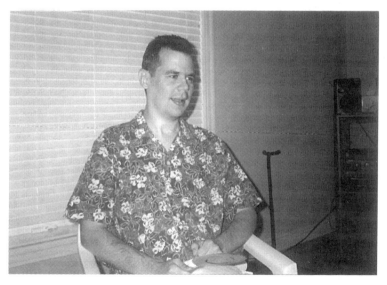

Kevin is conveying the feeling of *peaceful* to his therapist by gazing sweetly into her eyes.

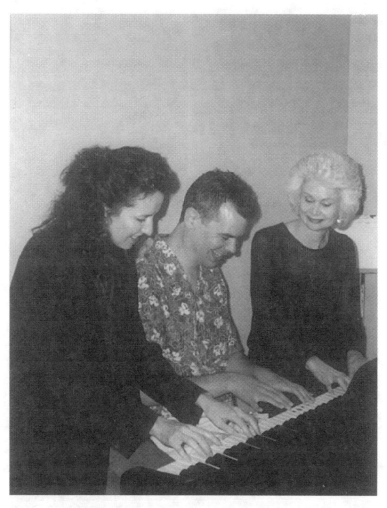

Kevin, Hope, and I are playing all white notes on the piano improvising to Kevin's lead. In this exciting activity Kevin is able to communicate and build confidence.

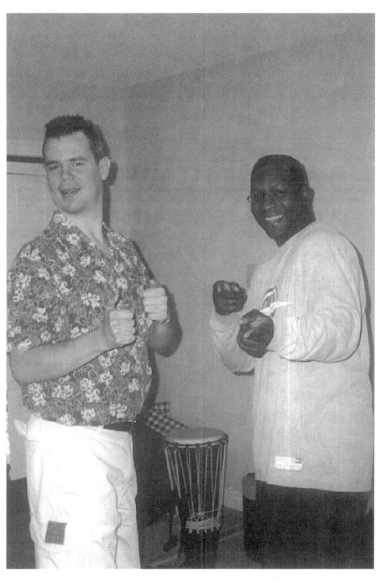

In therapy Kevin's dancing to lively music helps him to relate to Rodney, his group home manager. Activities using large motor movements energize him.

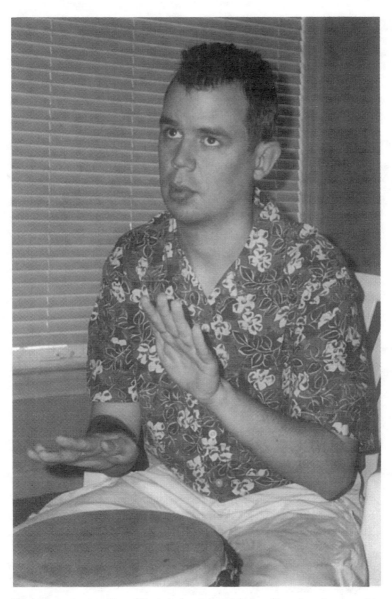

Drumming stimulates Kevin's brain and helps him to play out his TS symptoms and obsessive-compulsive behaviors.

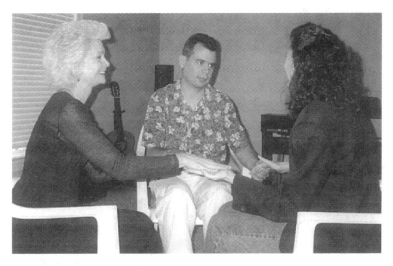

While listening to Enya's music, Kevin, Hope, and I are making circular hand movements to connect and create a feeling of safety.

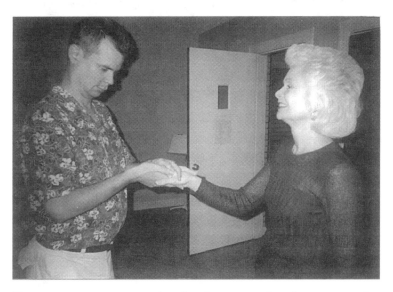

Kevin is nurturing me with a hand massage that demonstrates his gentle nature.

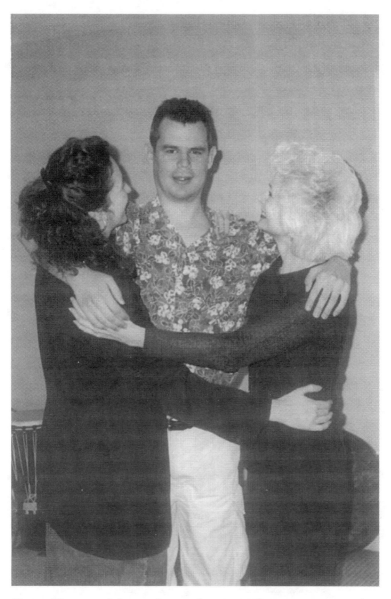

Kevin, Hope, and I are closing the music therapy session with a group hug.

After years of music therapy, Kevin has developed from a shy, withdrawn, and tense man into a happier, more talkative and relaxed person. Not only does he answer questions without hesitation, but he also takes the initiative to let us know what he needs. Since his memory has improved, he is more responsible about keeping track of his belongings. More noticeably, Kevin has fewer vocal tics and a longer attention span. Because of music therapy and the elimination of sodas, he has stopped running away from his group home.

Due to a weakness in his social development, Kevin has been practicing the basic greetings of *Hi* and *Bye* in his therapy sessions. Being more aware of others, he is less caught up in his head. Kevin used to live on "another planet" and tune out totally; now he is more "here." I make a habit of engaging him in informal conversation often, following the music therapist as a role-model.

I feel encouraged that music therapy is improving Kevin's cognitive abilities. When he spoke to me the other day at work, I barely recognized my son's voice. Since his voice sounded almost normal in affect for just a moment, it inspired me to believe that he was one step closer to normality.

Having witnessed Kevin's growth through music therapy, I believe that he can learn any task. This ability became evident when he quickly learned how to assemble a lamp while working at a hobby store. I commend Kevin for his patience with his learning process. If he can be patient, so can I. Patience is becoming my middle name—a gift that Kevin has given to me.

Kevin's bedroom is his music realm, where he listens to country western music on the radio and to heavy metal music on CDs. He is probably the only person on the planet who likes both country music and heavy metal! Rap music is stimulating to him, too.

Outside of therapy sessions, Kevin has been shy about singing in front of others. I have encouraged him to sing to me, and twice he has miraculously performed. He takes huge breaths to initiate the first words of his songs, and then his eyes light up when he sings. Expressing his own music stimulates him and livens him up.

On a recent drive to the country I was honored by Kevin's performance. After I sang wholeheartedly for fifteen minutes, I urged him to sing. I was shocked when he burst into a country western song; he even imitated the slurred inflection of a country western singer. When he stopped, I asked him for another round of song. He followed my cue of "one, two, three" for several rounds of singing until we reached our destination. To my delight, the car traumas of our past began to fade away during our fun trip filled with his easy-going country music.

Holidays have become great tests of Kevin's progress. I truly believe that his participation in music therapy has matured him to the point of being able to enjoy Christmas with ease. He was an angel when our family members came together last Christmas. We noticed how grown-up he had become. Instead of anxiously moving around the house or moping in a bed, as he had done in the past, he remained seated, relaxed, and open to conversation. For the first time, he actually related to my sister, who was visiting us from out-of-town.

Kevin and I will continue to bond at an even deeper level through mirroring, singing, listening to music, playing drums, and attending musical events. Last Christmas Eve, Kevin, Megan, and I attended a wonderful service at their father's beautiful church, where Dad played the organ and directed the choir for its holiday musical event. I smiled proudly at Kevin as he sat quietly beside me on good behavior. He was captivated by the powerful organ sounds and the tender notes of the harp.

As Kevin and I continue to create our own music therapy experiences in our everyday lives, I look forward to maturing with him. In appropriate settings I will use singing as a tool to override his Tourette symptoms. Hopefully, he will be more willing to sing for me in the future. We have taken music therapy out of the session room and into real life. Though music is absent in most of our interactions, we are applying the principles of music therapy and are growing in our ability to create safer interactions between us.

I believe that music therapy has provided an effective training and intervention for my son. It has trained him to listen more to his inner voice, to monitor his behavior, and to come out of his shell. Since control issues are inherent in the nature of Tourette syndrome (according to Hope), Kevin has learned to exercise better control by verbalizing his wants and needs. His improved behavior and language ability have demonstrated to me that music has a therapeutic, healing effect that would also benefit others with speech impairment, TS, and its related disorders of OCD, ADHD, and conduct disorder.

10

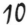

Will Work for Food!

During his twenty-sixth year, my son finally arrived at a point in his life when he was ready to manifest a part-time job. Utterly obsessed about finding employment, he wandered from his new day center to stores asking about jobs. Kevin's persistent demand, "I want a job!" persuaded the new employment specialist to make him a high priority for locating a job.

Before coming to the center, Kevin had spent four years attending a well-structured workshop, which gave him experience in doing tedious, repetitive tasks that developed small motor skills. Of course, his new staff at the center was unfamiliar with Kevin and didn't have any idea of his interests or capabilities. They soon discovered that he learned tasks easily while on the job and could do almost any work task in his typically perfectionistic manner.

Kevin's first job was busing tables at a fast-food restaurant. He demonstrated being a very careful, methodical worker, who learned to do the task correctly. He also began to watch out for drive thru traffic when taking trash bags to the dumpster. However, his staring at young female customers during work, as well as the soda cups left on the tables, became a major distraction. One day, he was caught sneaking carrot cake from the refrigerator. The cake was becoming the latest temptation for his sweet tooth.

Although the restaurant management was very tolerant of his lack of self-control, Kevin's group home staff decided to remove him from his job. They wanted to find a quieter work environment for him without the distraction of sodas and sweets. Over the course of eight months as a bus boy, he had learned his tasks well yet experienced some trouble staying on task. He tended to make long visits to the bathroom to let out his emotional outbursts. On occasion, he shocked customers during the lunch hour with some compulsive swearing.

Since Kevin's employment specialist was too busy to focus on finding him another job, my growing impatience motivated me to venture out and find one for him. As the mother of a son with a disability, everyone was sympathetic to my job search for him. After I showed the manager of a large hobby store a picture of Kevin, he consented to letting him work part-time. While marking prices on new merchandise with a pricing gun in the back stockroom, he was supervised by a job coach. His responsibilities also involved crushing boxes and assembling new lamps, which he quickly mastered.

Once again, Kevin got distracted during lunch in the break room, begging other employees for sodas. One fateful day, he impulsively ran through the store like a child, oblivious to customers milling around. As the story goes, he nearly ran down an elderly woman with a walker in front of his store manager, who couldn't control him. The customer's friend grabbed him by the arm and made him stop running. After his carefree dash through the store, Kevin was fired. His free-spirited nature had gotten the best of him!

I was livid and could not accept his firing. After forcing myself to go to the hobby store, I talked to several department managers about the episode and gathered first-hand information from their point of view. As a result, six female employees wrote letters on Kevin's behalf, believing that he was poorly supervised on the day of his firing. They were disturbed that he could no longer work in the store. I was terribly disappointed that his store manager did not give Kevin a second chance, but I figured his pride was hurt after he failed to stop him running. However, he did tell me that he feared Kevin would run again and hurt somebody.

Never giving up, I walked into a discount department store and found my son a job as a stockroom assistant. Right from the start, the store manager insisted that Kevin have ongoing supervision, and I consented. I worked with him for a few days until his former job coach arrived on the scene to assist him learning his new routine—hanging up juniors, misses, and men's shirts on different hangers and applying sensor tags to name-brand clothing. One day he goofed on a halter top and placed the sensor button in the middle of the front! While working there for many months, Kevin was distracted by the female staff who darted in and out of the stockroom. He once approached his favorite attraction, a petite manager with long silky hair, and blurted out with a flirting grin, "I am a dude!" Fortunately the young woman smiled and nodded kindly toward him.

Eventually, Kevin's job-coaching funds from the rehabilitation commission ran out, disallowing him to receive funding for supervision at work for two years. Knowing that he needed supervision, I faithfully volunteered to take on the responsibility of job-coaching him at the store. Though the manager never trained us, we worked steadily for three months as an efficient team: Kevin the whiz at tearing plastic wrapping off of new merchandise, and I the pro at rushing the clothing to its proper category on the long worktable.

Kevin and I loved the stimulation of the young girls buzzing around us, even though we usually spent long hours working by ourselves. One day Kevin zoomed off at lightning speed down the runway of the stockroom aisle and out the door into the main room. Fortunately, one of the male workers caught Kevin before he ran too far. Once again, my son created a stir and almost got fired, but the kind manager gave him a second chance when I told her that we would increase his medication dose.

One month later, the store management changed, and Kevin and I were abruptly asked to leave by a Human Resource officer. Apparently, the district manager, who hadn't known about Kevin, was shocked that a person with a disability was working there. I was traumatized by his rash decision and, as Kevin's mother, became irate. Though it was a tragic moment for me, I still remember how passionately I stood up for Kevin in front of the HR person. She reported to me that he was not working up to the standard of the other stockroom assistants. Yet, according to my observation, he worked more steadily than the other stockroom assistants, most of whom engaged in talking. The company policy was easy come, easy go. Poor Kevin! His lack of awareness about what had happened motivated me to find another job for him quickly.

After several weeks of searching through agencies, I contacted the main branch of the public library and found him a volunteer job on its top floor, far removed from the public. The volunteer coordinator was moved by a mother who was willing to work with a son with a disability. I remember thinking: *Wow! A job on an all-staff floor! He can't possibly run down the elevator. How perfect for Kevin. What luck, We've struck gold!*

When I picked Kevin up for work, he periodically tested me in the car with his favorite question, "Will you take me to the store and buy me a soda?" I asked him what the answer was, and he always said "no." Walking to the library together provided a great warm-up exercise for Kevin and me. On the way, he let off steam babbling in his own strange language. One of his quirky speech mannerisms involved speaking in polarities, such as, "You're my mother," and later, "You're not my mother." Or, he'd say, "I'm a baseball player," followed by, "I'm not a baseball player." He repeated the statements in an emphatic tone until he played them out.

For six months, Kevin and I succeeded in a short term job of unpacking brand-new books and sorting them alphabetically for circulation to branch libraries. Our work also entailed tearing off shrink wrap from video tapes and encyclopedias and removing covers from children's books. Though our tasks were tedious and tiring, we managed to get a great cardiovascular work-out and perform a service for the city at the same time. Kevin and I operated as a team, in which he was the hands and muscles and I the head and sorter. Teamwork motivated him more than working by himself. When he needed prodding, I told him to "keep on trucking." Pushing heavy book trucks was the name of the game! Since the aisles got so congested, our bumping into boxes or other book trucks was perfectly acceptable.

As a library volunteer, Kevin required frequent eye contact to maintain a connection with me during work, thus keeping him quiet and task-oriented. Otherwise, he escaped into staring at staff or sometimes chattering out loud to himself with a smile, "I'm being bad," or "I'm being good." I tended to leave him alone until his words would fizzle out. When he continued repeating with more volume, I intervened to redirect him. On some workdays, he giggled inappropriately or verbalized his random thoughts more freely. One of his typical expressions to me at work was, "I work here. You don't work here." He liked to distinguish between my role as the coach and his role as the worker.

Kevin's strength lay in following directions and knowing what to do with tools and boxes. Being agile and having a good balance kept him from dropping objects. He could manipulate scissors carefully while cutting the taped packaging that protected the new books. Being strong, he could carry heavy boxes or push weighty book trucks. Having excellent finger dexterity, he tirelessly tore shrink wrap off books and videos. Lining up new books or CDs perfectly helped him to work through his compulsive tendencies. Even though he was one-track minded, he learned to adjust to a second task easily.

Since Kevin didn't stand out with an obvious disability, his annoying behavior of staring in the workplace would confuse and catch people off guard. He had trouble containing his high energy level without my help. Part of my responsibility was to take him by the hand and redirect him from a potential behavioral clash with another person.

One day on the elevator, I saw him compulsively touch someone on the shoulder before I could grab his hand. After this episode, I realized I needed to sandwich myself between him and others and pay closer attention to his compulsive responses. Since I knew he loved making eyes at women on the elevator before saying something to them, I learned to distract him by giving him good eye contact and holding his arm. Being drawn to women and over-stimulated by their friendly presence, Kevin sometimes smiled or giggled too overtly at them.

My son has worked a variety of jobs and has successfully learned to do many different types of tasks. In his current volunteer job, he works with me around an all-male staff in the warehouse for the public library system, sorting books for circulation to its twenty branch libraries. It is tedious, repetitious work but very easy. After I pass the books to Kevin, he places them in the correct branch library bags. Sometimes I sing the name of the branch to him so that he can hear the word in his mind and memorize its location. Then he carries the heavy canvas bags filled with books to the proper branch bin for delivery. We often trade off; he passes books to me, and I put them in the appropriate branch bags.

Sometimes Kevin is not able to censor his thoughts at work and, therefore, has emotional outbursts. He might raise his voice and repeat, "Move, Patricia," or "Quit it!" if he perceives that I am too close to him. I will move either farther away or around the corner to interrupt his thought. Without me in front of his face, he will usually stop. Twice he has had a rage attack at his job after shouting, "White man is hurting me!" Whenever I sense he's becoming anxious, I divert him immediately by taking him to the water fountain, initiating a competitive speed game on a task, or having him phone staff.

My foremost thought is to remain calm. Sometimes, however, my son talks to himself and quietly makes statements that are based on truth, such as "I live at Pendleton group home," or "I am a man." His jabbering is his own form of therapy that keeps him grounded in reality on the job.

While job-coaching Kevin, I rely on my patience to communicate with him. First I slow down, then breathe, and sometimes count to five. Silence and intuition enable me to read his behavior easily. If he's focused, I give him instructions by using non-verbal cues.

During moments when Kevin shows disinterest in work, I exercise my authority by looking him straight in the eye and telling him, "I am the job coach, and you must work." If he doesn't respond favorably, I can invariably tempt him to keep on working by reminding him about dinner after work. Having an unfailing interest in food, he continues to stay on task or just take a short break.

Without a doubt, the way to my son's heart is through his stomach. Sharing dinner with me is Kevin's all-time favorite activity. If his behavior is inappropriate at the restaurant, I remind him immediately that he can choose to act appropriately or we will leave. His usual choice is to behave better and stay with me.

In spite of occasional behavioral problems, Kevin is able to work non-stop. It takes him less than an hour to warm up to his task. After getting on a roll, he works steadily without needing prompting or reassurance. He also responds extremely well to praise and frequent high fives.

In order to alleviate straining his back, I have coached him to learn to squat when unpacking a bag or box of books on the floor. Kevin demonstrates the neurological tendency of bending over called posturing when working or talking to someone at the site. Exhibiting a poor understanding of spatial relationships, he lacks the natural ability to position his body out of people's way. When working together, we build momentum by feeding off of each other's energy. Compensating for his handicap, I make up for his distractibility by role-modeling a rapid pace and a positive attitude. I challenge myself to surpass any expectations that our supervisor might have for us. Coaching Kevin is indeed a physical, mental, and spiritual work-out.

After years of being a methodical worker, Kevin's pace is beginning to pick up. Knowing what to expect helps him to work at a faster tempo and focus more on the job. A snack break with water also motivates him to stay on track and provides a structured rest period. Occasionally, Kevin cycles into a control game with me, but we work it out by taking a water break or having him sit and rest. Leaving him alone is usually the best medicine. Since he feels safe with me, he allows himself to do what he wants, and I continue to remain flexible to his mood swings and erratic nature.

Whenever I praise Kevin for doing a good job at work, I have the pleasure of seeing his radiant smile. He beams with pride and joy while exchanging high fives with me, knowing that he has earned his reward of going to dinner. Since he is so relaxed after working, I have concluded that carrying heavy bags is great exercise for him and sorting books helps him work out his compulsive tendencies.

Kevin has become a valuable worker and an asset to the public library system. In fact, our volunteer coordinator told us that his speediness in unpacking new books, from fifty to seventy boxes a day, helped the library to circulate books rapidly through the system to their branch libraries.

My greatest hope is that someday Kevin will be able to work at a job without supervision and that his occasional outbursts will subside over time with the help of experience and music therapy. I continue to visualize him in the future working by himself and staying on task. Most importantly, I want Kevin to thrive on his work with a passion and to move around on his own accord. I trust that working on a job will become an integral part of Kevin's being.

11

One Crazy Christmas

One Christmas Eve afternoon, I remember driving with Kevin to my mother's house for the holidays. Upon arriving, we found mother in bed and her nurse's aide drinking a soda in the kitchen. On an impulse, Kevin tried to grab the drink out of her hand and shocked the poor woman! For the rest of the day, my son eyed her every second, and she was too afraid to drink another soda.

During another Christmas visit, Kevin grabbed the tub of ice cream out of my mother's freezer and started digging into it. I quickly moved the ice cream to a neighbor's freezer. With the help of a friend, I coped with Kevin's frantic behavior by redirecting him through the mirroring technique that we had learned in music therapy. While seated opposite him in the living room, we let him be the leader and imitated his gestures helping him to control his impulsivity. At first, some of my relatives were staring at us, wondering what we were doing. Gradually, they began to understand our process, and some of them even joined us and mirrored his gestures back.

And so the mirroring process became one big crazy family affair. Kevin began to smile and laugh, and feeling more relaxed, he ate up the attention from everybody. As a result, we succeeded in communicating with him non-verbally and in relieving his anxiety.

Since the music therapy technique had a calming effect on Kevin's behavior, he began to settle in for our family Christmas event. I think Kevin's humor helped everybody to loosen up and enjoy the moment. The power of music therapy woke all of us out of our trance into the Christmas spirit of giggles and laughter.

At the end of our visit, Kevin asked my pretty blond-headed niece if she would "go" with him. When she sweetly declined his romantic invitation, he received her smile and compassion as a gift instead.

12

Reflections

Although my healing actually started when Kevin was born, I wasn't aware of it until I placed him in the hospital when he was ten. Later, during the years of coping with him as a teenager, I built a protective wall around me and isolated myself from my parents. Because Kevin consumed so much of my time, I lost many friends. Several of them were threatened by his strange disorder, and so was I.

When I reflect back to those challenging days in Kevin's life, I recall feeling very alone. Sometimes I burst into tears and pitied myself, *Why me? Why am I the mother of this crazy son? Why him? Why is his brain like this?* Hitting my fist on the pillow, I shouted, *This isn't fair! Why do I have to go through this alone?*

However, I wasn't always alone. When Kevin was sixteen, a male friend lived at my house for a short time and served as my bodyguard. Kevin saw him as strong and, in contrast, saw me as weak. My son's perception of me began to fuel his control over my life. Unfortunately, after four months, I asked my friend to leave because we weren't getting along.

On different occasions, several female friends formed a rescue squad and accompanied me in my car to track Kevin running on the road. To comfort me, another close friend distracted me on the phone during one of Kevin's banging fits on my bedroom door.

At one point, I organized a whole crew of friends who took turns sitting with Kevin whenever I needed to run errands or take an afternoon off. I also paid a few of them to supervise Kevin on a part-time basis while I did some light housekeeping. I became the CEO of Kevin Care, Inc!

Even though I endured many hectic spells with my son, I learned to seize the moment and tackle problems immediately to keep my life running. I became an expert juggler of time and an excellent problem-solver. I adamantly refused to go nuts because of Kevin. Nor would I let him get me down for more than a few days! I liked facing challenges, and Kevin certainly brought me more than my fair share.

Kevin's condition was so mysterious that I was constantly wondering what had gone awry. *Did something happen to him during childbirth? Did the forceps that bruised his head cause brain damage? Did the anesthesia affect his brain when his hernia was removed at three months? Was it the high fever after his baby shots?* When Kevin abruptly withdrew from breastfeeding at thirteen months after nursing so regularly, I wondered, *What could have caused the sudden change in his behavior?*

While Kevin was a six-year-old, he had a series of persistent ear infections. *Could the infections have contaminated his brain, precipitating Tourette syndrome?* I tormented myself unmercifully by ruminating on all the possibilities of an error in his early childhood. On a deeper level, I felt responsible for Kevin's inability to grow into an emotionally balanced child. I empathized with his emotional pain and discomfort with his

Tourette symptoms and also his trouble managing his high energy. Sometimes he just whimpered in sheer frustration.

After learning about the genetic factor of TS, I began to settle down and stop tormenting myself. So many questions haunted me for years until I decided that the cause didn't matter. Though I was making peace with my son's condition, some days I was gripped with the painful reality that I was the only person who was emotionally available for him. I was truly the mainstay in his life—the one who held his hand and kept him focused on everyday reality.

During many years of Kevin's life, I sincerely felt like a victim of his TS disorder. However, I eventually saw how he served me by bringing painful childhood memories to the surface and giving me a chance to heal on them. Having grown up with a domineering father, I fought against letting Kevin dominate my life and make me the prisoner that my father had. I began turning the victim pattern around during my process in music therapy. I could see past Kevin's physical symptoms and empower myself by sharing my feelings with him, even my hurt ones. As I became more detached from him, I experienced my son's pure, innocent heart.

Kevin's psychiatrist told me, when my son was ten, that he was uniquely different from other children, one in a million. I have been told the same about myself. Well-suited, Kevin and I are learning different lessons from each other. He's learning how to become more grounded in reality while I'm learning to trust God. Living most of the time on the edge of a crisis with Kevin, I believe divine presence is beside me every step of our way. I feel as though I am running in a never-ending marathon—as soon as I get a little comfortable, my son brings me another challenge that keeps me from resting on my laurels.

I now regard Kevin as an equal in our relationship, and through him I embrace opportunities to grow spiritually. In truth, he is the major healing agent in my life, who helps me to practice letting go and living in the moment. I am willing to do whatever is necessary to provide support and safety for him. Though I accept his Tourette syndrome condition as purposeful for our growth, I remain hopeful for improvement on his behavioral disability.

As a symptom of his Tourette disorder, Kevin has made strange comments about me to others through the years. For example, I recall some humorous remarks made during an extensive psychological test. According to the assessment, when asked about me, he jabbered that I was not his mother. He didn't know who I was. He said, "She's a hooker and sells dope." When asked "why?" he responded, "because she drives a fast sports car." Fortunately, I wasn't present during the testing, as his jabbering would have embarrassed me. At that time, I perceived him as unconsciously venting his anger and blaming me for his TS condition, but later I learned that his strange remarks exhibited the Tourette symptom of *coprolalia*.

Several times in the past, when Kevin became agitated, hungry, or unable to communicate his needs to me, he verbally abused me. This behavior typically occurred in the car. Sometimes he shouted at me, "Bitch, Bitch!" or screamed in my ear, "F%@# you!" Once, while riding with him on a local freeway, he yelled in my ear at least twenty times, "Stop it!" Unfortunately, giving him eye contact fueled stronger responses from him. Having learned my lesson, I silently kept my eyes on the road as he continued cursing at me. After such traumatic moments, I invariably needed several days to recover. I encouraged myself to regroup quickly in order to bounce back into our intense relationship.

Being a strong-willed person, I continue to confront the Tourette *intruder* inside Kevin, as well as the fearful parts inside me. Having endured many embarrassing, violent situations, I have learned to sense Kevin's volatility. As a result of these experiences, I use my head more and rely on my natural instincts. Feeling butterflies in my stomach forewarns me of an angry spell approaching or potential oppositional behavior. My warning signs prepare me to handle challenging situations by appealing to the calmest part inside me. I believe that I cannot calm Kevin down unless I am calm myself. Even though his emotional outbursts rarely occur now, I prevent those that do happen by being calm and swiftly redirecting him on the spot before they escalate. My emotional resilience has helped me heal myself, forgive Kevin, and carry on my life.

With the strongest intention, I have kept my life going without allowing Kevin's behavior to control me or throw me off my own path. For example, during the four years of taking care of Kevin at home, I continued teaching at the university. I only missed two days of work: one day while placing Kevin in the state hospital and another day while recovering from a major car wreck.

Granted, I was not a perfect person in the midst of Kevin's craziness. Some days I felt like a total wreck and cried my eyes out. My car accident was symbolic of my inner shattering, and somehow I got back on my feet and kept on trucking. One day, when the director of my teaching unit complimented me on my good mental health, I chuckled to myself because I was feeling frazzled at that time. She didn't even know that I was dealing with some of Kevin's heavy-duty behaviors. After each little trauma, I somehow managed to recover quickly, not allowing the stress to numb me out emotionally or cause physical problems.

In observing my son, I notice that every October and November he cycles into a period of extreme nervousness and compulsive running. For example, he might leave his day facility and run toward the highway nearby. Or he might take off running inside the video store on an outing with his class. During this specific time of year, Kevin requires stronger one-on-one supervision to prevent him from suddenly scaring strangers or even harming himself.

Whenever problems arise with Kevin at his home or day center, I make myself available for support to his staff. Having learned the value of teamwork, I know his staff needs my support as much as I need theirs. For example, one day when Kevin wouldn't budge from the bathroom floor at his day center, four teachers and I experimented with ways to get him to respond. When he wouldn't tell us what he needed, we realized Kevin was playing a control game. Sure enough, after we gave up and walked away, he got up on his own accord!

My bag of tools for coping with my son's inappropriate behaviors helps me to solve problems quickly. Having good self-discipline and time efficiency skills comes in handy for me. Never willing to give in to Kevin's weaknesses, I thrive on my own problem-solving ability to redirect him quickly and to encourage him to make healthy choices in the moment. For the most part, he can be redirected very easily.

Kevin is doing the best he can with his life, but he tends to act up when holding his feelings in or needing to be the center of attention. Very attuned to his intuition, he can pick up on intangibles that others do not detect. Whenever he blurts out words to someone, he might be seeing or sensing something that others are not aware of in themselves.

I am trusting the music therapy process to continue to promote Kevin's growth and to balance his brain chemistry. Kevin amuses me with his repetitious statements; sometimes, however, his loud voice can boom embarrassing remarks in public. I visualize that he will modulate his voice someday and will be able to tell me something only once instead of three or more times. I remind myself that, at least, Kevin is able to talk and his condition could be far worse.

After years of reflecting about our lives, I have concluded that Kevin himself is responsible for facing the lessons that his challenging life brings him. I have pondered the question, if this were his only lifetime, why would God deal him this hand? I have reconciled that Kevin's neurological condition must be a part of his own divine plan, in which I have been chosen to be a key player.

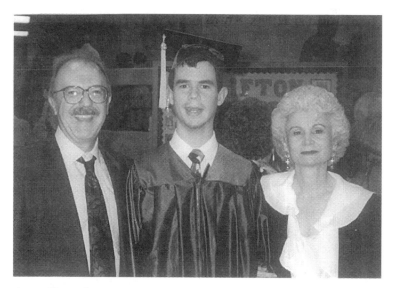

At 22 Kevin beams as a high school graduate while Mom and Dad are crying with joy that he has finally made it!

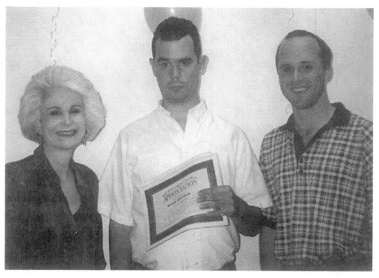

At 26 Kevin (with me and Brad Caffey) is awarded a Certificate of Appreciation for volunteer work at the Austin Humane Society.

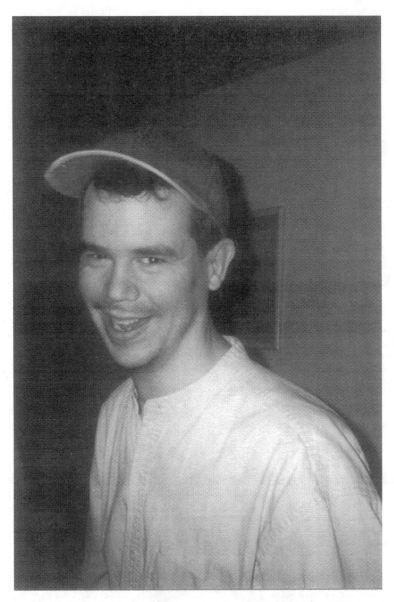

Celebrating his 28th birthday, Kevin shows the soothing effects of the drug Resperidal that has curbed his emotional outbursts.

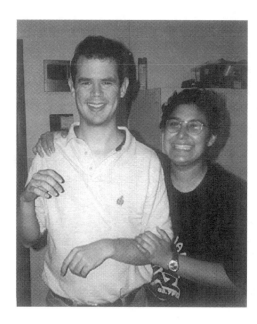

At 29 Kevin
giggles with
teacher Yvette
at his center.

Kev and Paul,
his housemate,
interact while
reading at
their center
in Austin, TX.

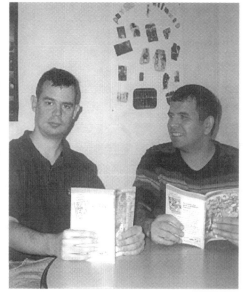

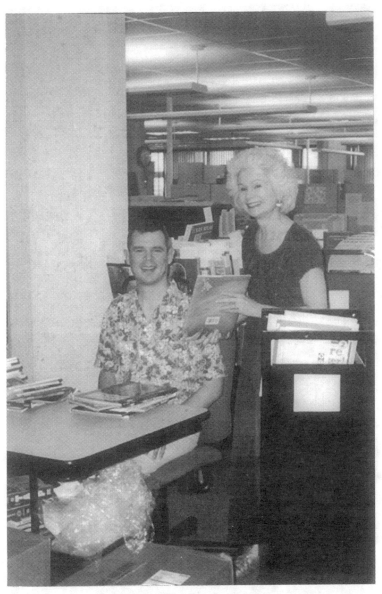

At our volunteer library job in 2000, Kevin and I are unpacking new children's books and removing their covers for processing.

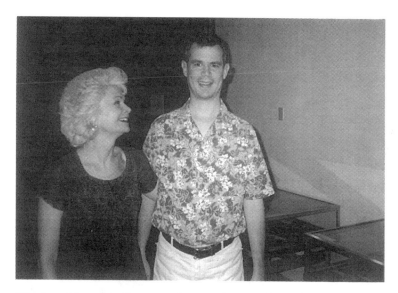

Tired and hungry after unpacking 50 boxes of library books, Kevin and I exchange high fives, waiting for the elevator to go to dinner.

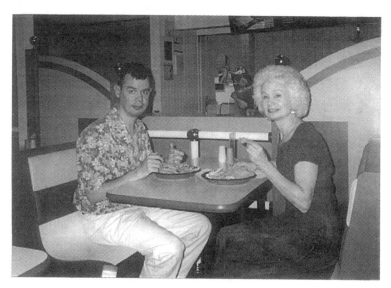

After working cooperatively at his job, Kevin is being rewarded at his favorite fast food restaurant.

13

Blessing in Disguise

Kevin was the baby that I had always dreamed of having—the one I feared I would never have. During the few years leading up to his birth, I faced an intense fear of dying that disappeared when I became pregnant with him. Later, in his difficult teens, I became fearful about living out the rest of my life with his TS. My fear dissipated, however, after gaining confidence in myself and an appreciation for Kevin's lively presence in my life. I began to see the light at the end of the tunnel in his big brown eyes. Behind the disguise of Tourette syndrome, I recognized his inner spirit as a blessing to me.

My parenting experiences have been uniquely different from other mothers—considerably more intense and time-consuming! I admit that Kevin takes the prize for being the most challenging yet loveable person in my life. My interactions with other people are certainly easier compared to those with him. In spite of difficulties with his behavior, I know he has a big heart. He shares his humor with me and, like a lightning bolt, jolts me into the moment. He is also a reminder to me that life has a natural ebb and flow from one extreme to the other—contracting and opening up. I am grateful to him for challenging me to be the most that I can be.

Kevin's unpredictable personality has followed me through life and conditioned me to handle other emergencies with courage and ease. Whenever his inappropriate behaviors appear, he brings me opportunities to let go and surrender. Over time, they pass and other behaviors show up. Music therapy taught me to ride through Kevin's roller coaster moments. Though sometimes afraid of his *intruder*, I've learned to stick it out, hold my ground, and keep my cool. I practice self-control and centering to cope with his sudden intrusive behaviors. I am usually able to detach myself emotionally from a trying situation, since I know that he tends to shift from a negative to a cooperative state. Learning how to be a neutral observer for a loved one with a disability is a powerful lesson and an opportunity to practice loving. Thank you, Kevin, for teaching me detachment!

The process of raising a son with a severe behavioral disability has motivated me to develop trust in my natural instincts. Recently, after Kevin yelled at me several times in the car, "Go! Go!" during a traffic jam, I broke into song to diffuse the energy of his outbursts. I made up words and a melody to express "go, go, go on the road through the traffic!" Luckily, the music interrupted his perseveration, and I was relieved that following my intuition had helped us out.

Since then, I have improvised with energetic singing while driving to redirect him and help me flow through his fits. If he shows distress in the car by shutting down, I may vocalize softly to a CD, in hopes of lulling him into a more open state. I've learned that improvising effectively alters his mood.

I'm embracing more parts of myself, including my vulnerabilities, while learning to accept Kevin's disorder freely and unconditionally. Being exposed to his neurological condition has helped me to appreciate my good mental health, along with my natural ability to express myself. Yet, after years of reality checks as his guardian, I have come to terms with my own limitations in dealing with his powerful disability. I can only handle Kevin with the help of medication, a group home, a complete staff, music therapy, and abundant prayers.

Due to the wide gaps in Kevin's development, he has had to learn everything through the help of others. Lacking communication skills, he depends on teachers to assist and give him direction. He demands respect from his helpers and expects them to be reasonable and clear. For example, he may ask me a question several times before he is satisfied that my response is a clear "yes" or "no." His adamant need for clarification has helped me to be as clear as possible, for I know very well that he will keep asking the same question until it's answered in a certain way. Honestly, I find his perseveration the most annoying TS symptom, but I am willing to meet the challenges of dealing with it.

Having Kevin in my life has brought me into the public eye without a doubt. Hanging out with an unusual son has helped me to forget about the social pretence of looking good around people. Being a lady was engrained in me by my mother during my childhood, but my son's outrageousness won't let me hide anymore. Before giving birth to him, I considered myself a very private person, who shied away from calling attention to myself. Though I'd rather be seen under different circumstances, I have accepted public exposure with him as a part of my life. I am learning to observe other people's reactions to him without taking them to heart.

Because I love and accept Kevin dearly, I like spending time with him regardless of his inappropriateness. He clearly knows I love him, and when told, he lights up like a light bulb. Refusing to let my fear of being embarrassed get in the way, I have made his neurological condition okay in my heart. On a positive note, Kevin is mainstreaming and receiving acceptance in the public through his job, in spite of his Tourette syndrome disorder. I am grateful that he truly loves being a part of the "normal" population, which mirrors back to him appropriate behaviors.

Our active non-verbal communication helps Kevin and me to stay bonded. By mimicking his movements to connect with him non-verbally, I adjust to Kevin's rhythm at work, just as I have practiced mirroring his gestures and tics in our music therapy sessions.

Because of his strength, I am motivated to stay physically fit—working out regularly and eating nutritiously. Throughout the years, Kevin and I have enjoyed playing racquetball and basketball, and even jogging and hiking together. Healthy living has become a wonderful by-product of keeping up with my athletic son.

Kevin's presence in my life has taught me to believe that all of life's experiences are purposeful. His tremendous impact on my path has resulted in one big healing crisis. As a catalyst, he has triggered the whole range of feelings in me— from disappointment to fear to childlike joy. I celebrate every little step my son makes as a major accomplishment in his development. I am proud that Kevin accepts "no" for an answer and can be redirected when he perseverates. I also honor my growth in having learned new ways to help him and to take care of myself. My calmness around him has transferred into other areas of my life, where I feel that I have become more compassionate but, at the same time, neutral and detached.

My persistent son challenges me by testing my firmness in being consistent with him. I am determined to hold the focus on his maturing emotionally, developing stronger self-control, and working more responsibly with his compulsive behaviors. Kevin is more responsive to me when I am gentle but firm. In the midst of his inappropriate behaviors, I am capable of remaining centered if I remember to pause for a moment and connect with my center.

My daughter Megan has matured greatly from growing up with a brother who has Tourette syndrome. After graduating from high school, she shared about her experience in a short essay: "I learned patience in helping Kevin to communicate. He was almost always very loving toward me and looked up to me because he wanted to be like me. I felt that I could communicate to him without words. I developed compassion for him and his disabled classmates and saw the beauty in these special people, who are truly our teachers for many great lessons." Megan continues to maintain a loving relationship with Kevin, and he perks up when she comes to visit him for the Christmas holidays.

Once in awhile, I feel the need for acknowledgement from Kevin. I fantasize that some day he will tell me how much he appreciates all the time I spend with him. Then I remember he is already acknowledging me by receiving my love and guidance. He knows that I'll never leave him and that it's safe for him to be himself. Wow, what trust he has in me!

Kevin symbolizes to me a vulnerable plant that had a strong beginning but needs loving attention in order to thrive. Though he doesn't bear fruit or bloom as rapidly as a healthy flowering plant, he continues to grow at his own rate to sustain himself. I nurture him and give him love, truly believing that my purpose in life is to give to him and that his purpose is to receive from me.

Because of our purpose together, Kevin and I are walking hand in hand until his independence day. I hope to let go of his hand when I trust him more to stay on track. Every step of our way, I keep in mind my goal of empowering him to become an independent, responsible person and myself to grow as a trusting, grateful human being.

14

Kevin: A Gift from Heaven

Throughout my son's life, I have learned to trust Kevin and God to take care of him. Knowing in my heart that I have little control over his actions, I have witnessed his ability to protect himself from physical and emotional harm. My son is so trusting of people and, despite his "You are devil" tic, sees others as all good and kind.

I believe Kevin has a sixth sense that supports him out in the world. One rainy night after midnight, he wandered the dark streets for several hours alone before returning to his group home in the early morning. Though his feet were bloody and sore from his long night out, he succeeded in finding his way home safely.

Over the years, Kevin has demonstrated a knack for manifesting positive experiences in his life. This inherent ability reassures me of his safety. One afternoon he ran away from his group home to a neighborhood on the other side of town and knocked on a stranger's door. Kevin harmlessly asked him for a soda. The elderly man made a friendly phone call to let me know my son was at his house. Kevin had found a welcoming door! While driving frantically to pick him up, I smiled to myself at the man's act of kindness. Unafraid of people, my son had drawn a safe circumstance to him. He must surely have a guardian angel watching over him!

Years ago during bouts of unsettling outbursts, I was able to maneuver and redirect Kevin intuitively. However, one fearful day after all maneuvers failed, I had to rely on my faith. In that suspended moment when I saw Kevin preparing to grab my throat, I experienced my vulnerability as a human being. Standing in the dining room at the peak of his rage, I prayerfully asked for protection. In terror, I surrendered my urge to defend myself, and so did he. Miraculously, he backed off and stood quietly at arms' length. He had transformed into a peaceful human being.

After that day, I began to trust that I would not have to endure difficulties with Kevin alone. I believed that I had a guardian angel protecting me. Whenever I asked for spiritual help, I felt its presence. Even today, I welcome spiritual assistance in all matters with Kevin.

My deep-seated love for Kevin is the single most motivating force that allows me to be with him. Music therapy has helped me to access the strong love I have for him, beneath the fear of his harming me. He teaches me to love unconditionally. His gift from heaven is loving—the key to our hearts.

Epilogue

Though my story conveys today's truth about Kevin and me, tomorrow will tell a different story. The unpredictable nature of TS will continue to create new experiences and challenging behaviors. Taking deep breaths, I walk along the rocky road of Tourette syndrome. My journey with Kevin will bring me healing opportunities that carve new chapters into my life.

In reading my memoir, you have witnessed the inside story of a mother who doesn't give up. Living faithfully day after day on the edge with Kevin is a continual process of praying to God and relying on His stamina to roll with life's punches. Kevin's imbalanced moments have tested my strength and integrity. Just as the pendulum of life swings from negative to positive, his behavior shifts from oppositional to cooperative. On days when I feel like resigning from motherhood, my spiritual side pulls me back in the ring.

While writing, I have struggled with words and emotions, pouring out my heart in hopes of helping you in some way. I send blessings to each of you along your path, inviting you to cope from your loving heart and to explore music therapy for you and your loved ones with TS and other disorders.

Q & A about Music Therapy

What is music therapy?

Music therapy utilizes music as a means to affect physiological, psychological, and emotional responses in individual clients. It will also lessen their dependency on pharmaceutical and hospitalized care.

What do music therapists do?

Music therapists assess emotional well-being, physical health, social functioning, communication abilities, and cognitive skills through musical responses. Designing sessions based on client needs, the therapists make use of music improvisation, receptive listening, and musical performance. In compliance with the standards of the American Music Therapy Association and the certification board for music therapists, they participate in treatment planning, ongoing evaluation, and follow-up.

Where do music therapists work?

The therapists provide services in hospitals, rehabilitative and correctional facilities, outpatient clinics, day care treatment centers, agencies for disabled persons, mental health centers, halfway houses, and schools.

How is music therapy utilized in schools?

Schools hire music therapists to provide music therapy services listed on the Individualized Education Plan for mainstreamed special students. Music learning strengthens communication and coordination skills.

What is a typical music therapy session like?

The session is based on the client's treatment plan and supports different types of needs.

Do I need musical talent to benefit from music therapy?

No, everyone can benefit from music therapy.

What is the history of music therapy as a profession?

The idea of music as a healing influence reflects back to the writings of Aristotle and Plato. Modern music therapy began after World War I and II when community musicians went to hospitals to perform for the veterans, who were suffering from physical and emotional trauma. After the patients showed remarkable physical and emotional responses to music, the hospitals wanted to hire therapeutically trained musicians. In 1944 the first music therapy degree program in the world was founded at Michigan State University. At the present time, sixty-nine American universities teach music therapy in their music school departments.

How can I locate a music therapist in my city?

For a list of music therapists in your city, please send your postal address via email: findMT@musictherapy.org
or via regular mail:
American Music Therapy Association, Inc
8455 Colesville Road, Suite 1000
Silver Spring, Maryland 20910
Phone (301) 589-3300 Fax (301) 589-5175

Resources

<u>Tourette Syndrome and Human Behavior</u>
David E. Comings, M.D., Hope Press, Duarte, CA, 1990
Hope Press (800) 321-4039 Fax (626) 358-3520
http://www.hopepress.com

Organizations

For information about Tourette syndrome, you can contact the following organizations:

Tourette Syndrome Association
42-50 Bell Boulevard
Suite 205
Bayside, NY 11361
(718) 224-2999 (888) 486-8738
http://tsa.mgh.harvard.edu

OC Foundation, Inc
337 Notch Hill Road
North Branford, CT 06471
(203) 315-2190 Fax (203) 315-2196
http://www.ocfoundation.org

Children and Adults with Attention Deficit Disorders
(CH.A.D.D.)
8181 Professional
Suite 201
Landover, MD 20785
(800) 233-4050 Fax (301) 396-7090
http://www.chadd.org